Jay A. Goldstein, MD

Chronic Fatigue Syndromes:
THE LIMBIC HYPOTHESIS

Pre-publication
REVIEWS,
COMMENTARIES,
EVALUATIONS . . .

"**D**R. Goldstein's encyclopedic grasp of biobehavioral and biomedical sciences arrives at a truly integrative theory of the complex pathophysiology of the chronic fatigue syndromes . . . .

Utilizing principles of psychoneuroimmunology . . . he arrives at dysfunction of that portion of the brain concerned with memory, emotions, sleep, stress responses, and regulation of endocrine and immune functions. . . . [This book] creatively offers a new model by which to understand this baffling condition."

George Freeman Solomon, MD
Professor of Psychiatry &
Biobehavioral Sciences, UCLA
& Chief, Psychoneuroimmunology
VA Medical Center, Sepulveda, CA

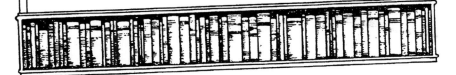

"**M**uch more than a hypothesis . . . [this book] is a comprehensive thesis which clearly defines the biological basis for many of the varied symptoms experienced by chronic fatigue symptom patients, as well as providing a rationale for the use of symptomatic therapies that have worked in many CFS patients . . . .

This volume chronicles the pioneering efforts of Dr. Jay Goldstein toward establishing chronic fatigue syndromes (CFS) as primary neurological disorders. Defying the conventional boundaries that separate neurology, psychiatry, and immunology, Dr. Goldstein has pursued an interdisciplinary approach to derive his unique understanding of CFS. His limbic hypothesis is based on extensive clinical observations and on the judicious testing of various drugs.

[The book] displays the breadth of Dr. Goldstein's understanding of the human nervous system and the role of the limbic system in integrating and regulating numerous neuropsychological functions. The presumed role of various hormones, neurotransmitter substances and immunologically acting and/or derived cytokines in limbic function is intelligently discussed. Dysregulation of these factors, as a result of persistent viral infections or other causes, could cause a tilting of the delicate balance of such critical physiological functions as sleep, fatigue, and memory, and could well result in the wide variety of symptoms and signs seen in CFS patients. The multiple actions of interleukin 1, within both the immune system and the nervous system, are detailed along with evidence of a possible impaired response to this critical cytokine in CFS patients. The book expands on the uses of modern radiological, laboratory, and cognitive-based testing methods which provide additional data on the neurological dysruptions typical of CFS patients.

Dr. Goldstein has provided the medical profession with a valuable handbook to assist in the diagnosis and treatment of the many patients afflicted with this devastating illness."

W. John Martin, MD, PhD
Professor of Pathology
University of Southern California
School of Medicine
Los Angeles, California

The Haworth Library of the Medical Neurobiology of Somatic Disorders

neuroimmunoendocrine networks in health & illness

Volume I: *Chronic Fatigue Syndromes: The Limbic Hypothesis*

Editor-in-Chief

Jay A. Goldstein, MD, Director
Chronic Fatigue Syndrome Institute, Anaheim, California

Advisory Board

Chronic Fatigue Syndromes

The Limbic Hypothesis

This volume is dedicated to those researchers and theorists who have inspired me in my search for the origins of Chronic Fatigue Syndrome:

George F. Solomon, MD

W. John Martin, MD, PhD

Ismael Mena, MD

Special appreciation for words of encouragement, editing of material, and critiques of earlier manuscripts goes to:

my wife, Gail Coplin Goldstein, EdD

Bill Cohen, Publisher of The Haworth Press, Inc.

Chronic Fatigue Syndromes
The Limbic Hypothesis

Jay A. Goldstein, MD

The Haworth Medical Press
An Imprint of The Haworth Press, Inc.
New York • London • Norwood (Australia)

Published by The Haworth Medical Press, Inc., an imprint of The Haworth Press, Inc., 10 Alice Street, Binghamton, NY 13904-1580

DISCLAIMER
Medicine is an ever-changing science. As new research and clinical experience broaden our knowledge, changes in treatment and drug therapy are required. While many suggestions for drug usages are made herein, the book is intended for educational purposes only, and the author, editor, and publisher do not accept liability in the event of negative consequences incurred as a result of information presented in this book. We do not claim that this information is necessarily accurate by the rigid, scientific standard applied for medical proof, and therefore make no warranty, express or implied, with respect to the material herein contained. Therefore the patient is urged to consult his or her own physician prior to following a course of treatment. The physician is urged to check the product information sheet included in the package of each drug he or she plans to administer to be certain the protocol followed is not in conflict with the manufacturer's inserts. When a discrepancy arises between these inserts and information in this book, the physician is encouraged to use his or her best professional judgement.

Figure 2 is reproduced with permission from the "British Medical Journal," September 26, 1992, Vol. 305.
Figure 3 is reproduced with permission from "The Biological Basis of Learning and Individuality" by Eric Kandel and Robert Hawkins. Copyright © 1992 by Scientific American, Inc.

Library of Congress Cataloging-in-Publication Data

Goldstein, Jay A.
    Chronic fatigue syndromes : the limbic hypothesis / Jay A. Goldstein.
      p.   cm.
    Includes bibliographical references and index.
    ISBN 1-56024-904-8 (alk. paper).
    1. Chronic fatigue syndrome. 2. Psychoneuroimmunology. 3. Limbic system. I. Title.
    [DNLM: 1. Fatigue Syndrome, Chronic. 2. Limbic System–physiopathology. WL 351 G624c]
RB150.F37G65   1992
616'.047–dc20
DNLM/DLC
for Library of Congress   92-48706
                                                         CIP

Series title: The Haworth Library of the Medical Neurobiology of Somatic Disorders: *neuroimmunoendocrine networks in health & illness*.

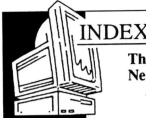

INDEXING & ABSTRACTING

The Haworth Library of the Medical Neurobiology of Somatic Disorders
neuroimmunoendocrine networks in health & illness

Articles/chapters in this publication are selectively indexed or abstracted in the following services as of the cover date of this volume:

- *Behavioral Medicine Abstracts,* The Society of Behavioral Medicine, 103 South Adams Street, Rockville, MD 20850

- *Biostatistica,* Executive Sciences Institute, 1005 Mississippi Avenue, Davenport, IA 52803

- *Digest of Neurology and Psychiatry,* The Institute of Living, 400 Washington Street, Hartford, CT 06106

- *Family Violence & Sexual Assault Bulletin,* Family Violence & Sexual Assault Institute, 1310 Clinic Drive, Tyler, TX 75701

- *General Science Index,* The H.W. Wilson Company, 950 University Avenue, Bronx, NY 10452

- *Oncology Information Service,* Leeds University, Leeds LS2 9JT England

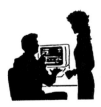

ABOUT THE AUTHOR

Jay A. Goldstein, MD, is Director of the Chronic Fatigue Syndrome Institutes in Anaheim and Santa Monica, California where he has seen over 3,000 CFS patients. He is Senior Editor for The Haworth Medical Press, the medical imprimatur of The Haworth Press, Inc.

Dr. Goldstein's current interest is concentrated on chronic fatigue syndrome. He is a Medical Advisor and regular contributor to *The CFIDS Chronicle* and the *CFIDS Chronicle Physician's Forum,* both published for the 20,000 plus members of the CFIDS Association, the largest and most important nonprofit charitable organization devoted to assisting chronic fatigue syndrome research and advocacy efforts.

Dr. Goldstein is Advisory Editor for the new *Journal of the Chronic Fatigue Syndromes,* also published by The Haworth Medical Press under the Editorship of Nancy Klimas, MD, Director of both the Chronic Fatigue Program and AIDS Program of the University of Miami Medical Center.

Dr. Goldstein's clinical studies include the application of brain mapping and brain functional imaging to CFS. He is the founder of the Southern California Chronic Fatigue Syndrome Study Group, a network of CFS researchers and clinicians, which include world-re-knowned researchers and academics from several southern California medical schools.

Dr. Goldstein's community outreach work includes the organization of an annual research conference that presents a different aspect of chronic fatigue syndrome each year. This year's title is the *Medical Neurobiology of Chronic Fatigue Syndrome and Fibromyalgia.*

Dr. Goldstein is Editor-in-Chief of *The Haworth Library of the Medical Neurobiology of Somatic Disorders: Neuroimmunoendocrine Networks in Health & Illness,* a peer-reviewed monograph series. Each volume in this new serial publication is co-published in both hardcover and softcover format in Haworth's new *DocuSerial*™ professional publishing program.

CONTENTS

Preface

This book is not intended to be a compilation of empirical research, although it is based on novel interpretations of previous research and newly acquired data. Nor is it primarily a presentation of my own clinical treatment trials, although I do refer to them. Rather, this book was written to consolidate and share my interpretations of the enigmatic disorder known as chronic fatigue syndrome (CFS).

As a clinician who diagnoses and treats patients with CFS, it has been important for me to develop and share with colleagues a rational concept of CFS pathophysiology from which symptoms would present themselves as derangements of normal regulatory mechanisms. In order to explain symptom generation, it has been necessary to integrate diverse areas of basic and clinical literature to prepare the foundations for rational therapeutic interventions. I am hopeful that this approach, and the etiologic suggestions that resulted, will be useful both to clinicians attempting to understand and help their CFS patients and to researchers who are investigating CFS in controlled experimental conditions.

Chronic fatigue syndrome represents, in my view, one of the most beleaguered segments of medicine. Its heroes and heroines, among both physicians and patients, are too numerous to list and credit properly in this short preface. But without the efforts of others cited throughout the text, this book could not have been brought into being.

My interest in the disease began in 1984, and since 1988 I have treated patients with CFS and related disorders almost exclusively. In the *CFIDS Chronicle*, an important journal for both CFS patients and their health care providers, I have presented continually refined concepts about CFS in the column entitled "The Evolving Hypothesis."

Positive feedback from colleagues about this column has encouraged me to consolidate into one book a point of view about CFS that could not be published within the page limit constraints of a single journal article. In order to prepare this work under the critical perspective of peer review, a small group of CFS researchers and clinicians agreed to provide evaluations. After three drafts a final version of this text was completed that was acceptable to both this peer group and the Editors of The Haworth Medical Press. I am grateful to my colleagues: an acceptable manuscript without their input and guidance would not have been possible. Portions of their final commentaries are printed in a different section of this text.

During the past decade, I hope my own role in CFS treatment and research has helped others by suggesting new hypotheses and synthesizing pertinent literature based on a long-term study of neurobiology and the regulation of bodily functions. CFS appears to be one of the most treatment-resistant disorders physicians encounter in primary care. I am hopeful that my own residency training in psychiatry and family medicine provided the eclectic perspective needed for specializing in CFS, which I view as a disorder of regulatory physiology.

The subtitle of this book underscores a vigorous caution that the hypothesis presented requires testing. I have been fortunate to be collaborating with researchers in academic medicine. We, as a group, have presented our work at numerous CFS conferences and have submitted manuscripts to scientific journals.

I hope that this book will stimulate readers to include evaluations of these medical hypotheses in their involvement with CFS. Perhaps its inferential model for CFS will suggest new ways to think about physiology in general, its alteration by disease, and new treatments based on these explorations.

My greatest satisfaction would be that the hypotheses presented herein prove to have sufficient heuristic value to initiate subsequent stages of scientific examination, and that some of the many dedicated scientists working in CFS research will be able to selectively transform hypothesis into postulate.

Jay A. Goldstein, MD, Director
Chronic Fatigue Syndrome Institute
Anaheim Hills, California

Introduction

When a thing was new, people said, "It is not true." Later, when the truth became obvious, people said, "Anyway, it is not important." And when its importance could not be denied, people said, "Anyway, it is not new."

–William James, 1842-1910

SUMMARY. Prior concepts and interpretations of chronic fatigue syndrome (CFS) from observations in clinical practice are noted and reviewed, starting with work on the treatment of acute infectious mononucleosis with H-2 blockers. The evolving hypotheses included consideration of the Epstein-Barr virus, cytokine dysregulation, and blocking H-2 receptors on suppressor-cytotoxic T-cells. The rapid effect of selected therapeutic agents on a percentage of patients suggested that in symptom generation neuroimmunoendocrine dysregulation was involved. Early work of Dr. Paul Cheney, Dr. Daniel Peterson, and Dr. John Martin is noted. A CFS symptom checklist is presented, and advances in research leading up to the limbic dysfunction hypothesis are discussed.

During the six years or so that I have been intensely interested in chronic fatigue syndrome (CFS), my understanding of the illness has undergone continued evolution. I originally conceived of CFS as being a disorder of inappropriate immune activation with the

[DocuSerial™ co-indexing entry]

"Introduction," Goldstein, J.A. Published in: *Haworth Library of the Medical Neurobiology of Somatic Disorders* (The Haworth Medical Press), Volume 1, 1993 and *Chronic Fatigue Syndromes: The Limbic Hypothesis,* Goldstein, J.A., The Haworth Medical Press, 1993.

symptoms caused by generation of immune transmitter substances called *cytokines*. I developed this concept from earlier work on the treatment of acute infectious mononucleosis with H-2 blockers, the results of which I published in 1981 and 1983.[1,2] Mononucleosis had been discovered to be caused by the Epstein-Barr virus (EBV) and it was known at the time that there was an elevated number of OKT8+ cells, now called suppressor/cytotoxic, or CD8+, cells. Although the symptoms were systemic and constitutional, and included fatigue, sore throat and obvious tonsillitis with enlarged lymph nodes and enlarged spleen, the Epstein-Barr virus could be recovered from only a few locations, such as the oropharynx. It seemed rather obvious that most of the signs and symptoms were caused by the reaction of the immune system to the virus, rather than the virus itself. Having a background in psychopharmacology, in which the study of transmitter-receptor interactions was fairly advanced, I reasoned that the OKT8+ lymphocytes might be producing a factor that was causing the syndrome. Cytokines or lymphokines were not well known yet, and the idea that cytokine dysregulation could cause disease was novel.

It had recently been discovered that suppressor T-cells had H-2 receptors on their cell membranes. I hoped that blocking these receptors might ameliorate infectious mononucleosis. Using cimetidine (Tagamet) and, later, ranitidine (Zantac), I was able to make most of my patients with mononucleosis feel normal within days, sometimes within hours. Their tonsillitis and enlarged lymph nodes resolved, too. This treatment did not work in every case, especially those in which unusual complications of mononucleosis, such as myocarditis, were present. The only way that I could understand the rapidity of this therapeutic effect was by postulating a decrease in the release of a suppressor/cytotoxic T-lymphocyte factor secreted by these cells when they were exposed to the Epstein-Barr virus. There must have been a genetic reason that some patients responded this way to the Epstein-Barr virus, or else almost everyone would get mononucleosis, since we are all exposed to the virus and develop antibodies to it. Africans appear to have different types of exposure, since they are more likely to get Burkitt's lymphoma and nasopharyngeal carcinoma, also caused by Epstein-Barr virus. Perhaps there are cofactors in Africa not present in developed nations.

One of these may be Euphorbia, a plant that produces phorbol esters, which are oncogenic by virtue of stimulation of protein kinase C. Tung oil present in sealants and varnishes is made from Euphorbia and has been proposed as a causative agent for chronic fatigue syndrome. Protein kinase C also produces long-term depression of synaptic efficiency and may be implicated in the encephalopathy of CFS.[3]

When CFS was described in the mid-1980s in the United States, the disorder was thought to be caused by the Epstein-Barr virus. I tried numerous patients on H-2 blockers who had "chronic Epstein-Barr virus disease" and about 20% of them improved rather remarkably, in a rapid manner reminiscent of my patients with infectious mononucleosis.[4] I did not know at that time that histamine acted at the H-2 receptor to enhance interleukin-1 (IL-1)-induced IL-1 gene expression and synthesis. I also did not know that it modulated the activity of several other neurotransmitters, including serotonin, and was involved in the stress response.[5] Serum levels of histidine, a histamine precursor, and tryptophan, a serotonin precursor, are low in fibromyalgia patients.[6] Histamine has been found to have a depressive effect on behavior, and this effect can be localized to the ventral hippocampus in rats. This effect may be mediated through the preoptic area and can be blocked by histamine antagonists injected into the ipsilateral hippocampus.[7] By 1987, experience had accumulated using alpha interferon and interleukin-2 for various disorders such as hepatitis and cancer, and a syndrome resembling CFS was often produced as an adverse reaction. Cognitive dysfunction was particularly prominent, and was the side effect most often causing termination of the therapy. I presented my hypothesis that CFS was a cytokine-induced disorder at a conference in Portland in 1987.[8]

By the time there was a symposium in Rhode Island in 1988,[9] I had formulated a five-stage hypothesis of disease etiology that I believe is still valid. I have outlined it in a series of articles in the *CFIDS Chronicle* called "The Evolving Hypothesis," and also presented it in a book, *Chronic Fatigue Syndrome: The Struggle for Health*, published in early 1990.[10] Briefly, I postulated that a latent predisposition (perhaps viral) to develop CFS was triggered by another agent. There then could be abnormal antigen processing and presentation, with inappropriate, or chronic, immune activation and generation of cytokines which could affect many organs. I believed the nervous system, especially the brain, to be most involved, and pictured it producing its own transmitter substances which would feed back to the immune system as well as to the rest of the body. I was influenced in this work by the research on bidirectional communication between the immune system and CNS by Edwin Blalock[11] and the concept of a psychosomatic network described by Candace Pert.[12] It was also apparent that chronic fatigue syndrome was a psychoneuroimmunologic disease since neurologic symptoms were so prominent and the severity of the illness, including flu-like symptoms, was so influenced by stress.

During 1987-89 I did lab tests that I thought would be relevant in order to understand the pathophysiology of the illness. All cytokines which could be measured at the time were studied, and only elevations in alpha interferon and interleukin-2 were found in certain patients. For numerous reasons (discussed in my previous book) I thought transforming growth factor-beta (TGF-beta) a likely candidate, but measuring it proved to be quite difficult, and techniques to measure its mRNA by the polymerase chain reaction, a nucleic acid amplification technique, had not been developed sufficiently for clinical use. I worked with Michael Palladino at Genentech for about a year on this project, with inconclusive results due to technical problems with the assay.

Several of us studying CFS in the mid-1980s were looking for a causative agent, probably a virus, since we were struck by the fact that there was often an acute flu-like onset, the illness sometimes seemed to occur in families, and there may have been some clustering in outbreaks. Numerous candidate microbes were (and are still) being studied. These included EBV, cytomegalovirus (CMV), human herpesvirus-6 (HHV-6), various enteroviruses, lentiviruses, candida, obscure mycoplasmas, and other retroviruses. The latter agents were attractive to me, as they were to Paul Cheney, who, along with Daniel Peterson, described a cluster of CFS cases in Incline Village, Nevada in 1984-85. We thought that a retrovirus could be latent in the immune system and/or brain, to be activated by various triggering stimuli such as other infectious agents, severe physical or emotional stress, surgery, childbirth, toxic agents, or sleep deprivation. This putative retrovirus, dubbed "Agent X," could even be transmitted through conception by DNA in the sperm or ovum, and might not manifest itself until many years later. Such a hypothesis has not been disproved, but is unlikely. The idea that CFS might have a single cause is seductive, particularly if it is regarded as a new illness (there is, however, good evidence for its existing in the earlier years of the twentieth century, and perhaps before).[13,14] I am frequently reminded of the assertion by the noted scientist and writer Lewis Thomas, paraphrased in *Virus Hunting,* by the virologist Robert Gallo: "multi-factor is multi-ignorance."[15]

In early 1988 I teamed up with Dr. John Martin, head of the Division of Molecular Pathology at the University of Southern California School of Medicine, and one of the developers of the polymerase chain reaction (PCR) technique. Dr. Martin started looking for the causative virus in my patients. Early results were promising, but isolation of "Agent X" proved elusive. Several centers have preliminary evidence of an "Agent X" and it remains to be seen whether they are all the same virus or whether sampling criteria or methodologies of virus isolation may have resulted in false positive results by some investigators. The implications of a viral etiology would be profound, not just for CFS but for much of medical practice, since so many neuropsychiatric, allergic, neuroen-docrine, psychosomatic, and functional disorders can be found in the CFS population. Symptoms of multi-system dysregulation frequently encountered in CFS patients are described in the following checklist. Their pathophysiology will be discussed subsequently.

CFS SYMPTOM CHECKLIST

This symptom checklist is not sufficient to diagnose Chronic Fatigue Syndrome unless other disorders have been ruled out by appropriate assessment.

A. Did your illness begin: *Sept. 1989*

     ☒ abruptly   ☐ gradually

     ☐ at what age? __43__   ☐ age now? __52__

B. Did your illness begin with a flu-like episode?

     ☒ yes   ☐ no

If yes: were lab tests done? _just normal blood work_

what tests? _CBC, Thyroid, adrenal function, immune system_

were abnormalities found? _No Thyroid + Central V Natural Killer Cells_

C. Were you treated for psychological problems prior to the onset of this illness?

     ☐ yes   ☒ no

        If yes: psychotherapy? ☐ yes   ☐ no

        medication _____

D. Did your illness follow exposure to new carpet/paint, tung oil, industrial solvents, pesticides, or other environmental toxins?

     ☐ yes   ☒ no

If yes, please describe: _____

E. Were you subject to prolonged stressors during childhood (e.g., abusive or dysfunctional home)?

     ☒ yes   ☐ no

If yes, please describe: _physical needs met but neglected emotionally - never touched, hugged, told "I love you" - only talked to when asked to do something. Stuffed a lot of feelings in. was shy & a loner._

F. Were you subject to unusual or extreme stressors in your life immediately prior to the onset of illness?

☒ yes   ☐ no

If yes, please describe: *I filed for divorce, started a new job & started graduate school all in Jan. of '89.*

G. Have you had silicone breast implants?

☒ yes   ☐ no

Have you had silicone injections?

☐ yes   ☐ no

Have you had collagen injections?

☐ yes   ☐ no

If yes to any of the above, did you have these procedures before or after the onset of your CFS symptoms?

☒ before   ☐ after

H. Are your symptoms worse: *I feel better when I'm warm!*

☐ in the summer   ☒ in the winter   ☐ no difference

I still have all the symptoms but am less likely to get an acute infection ... of everything in summer

Rate the severity of your symptoms from 0 to 10.

1. _8_   Fatigue–usually made worse by physical exercise

      Is your level of activity less than 50% of normal? ☒ yes ☐ no

2. ____   Cognitive function problems

      ✓   a. attention deficit disorder, including concentration problems

      ✓   b. calculation difficulties

I forget what I'm doing — put something in store room, etc. of refrigerator.

      (describe) *will add instead of subtract — think I'm doing it right but checkbook balance is always off —*

I feel like too much data is coming at me all — I can't slow my mind down to focus on anything — Being in a big new city in everything — I can't drive

CHRONIC FATIGUE SYNDROMES

    c. memory disturbance

    (describe)

    d. spatial disorientation, getting lost in familiar
       locations, problems judging distances

    e. frequently saying the wrong word

3.____ Psychological problems

    a. depression

    b. anxiety, which may include panic attacks and
       phobias (irrational fears)

    c. personality changes, usually a worsening of a
       previous mild tendency

    d. emotional lability (mood swings)

    e. psychosis

4.____ Other nervous system problems

    a. sleep disturbance

    b. headaches

    c. changes in visual acuity

    d. seizures

    e. numb or tingling feelings

    f. lightheadedness, feeling "spaced out"

    g. dysequilibrium

    h. frequent unusual nightmares

    i. difficulty moving your tongue to speak

    j. ringing in ears

    k. paralysis

    l. severe muscular weakness

    ✓ m. blackouts *– especially during*

    ✓ n. intolerance of bright lights

    ✓ o. intolerance of alcohol - *homeopathic drops*

    ____ p. alteration of taste, smell, and hearing

    ✓ q. non-restorative sleep

    ✓ r. decreased libido

    ✓ s. twitching muscles ("benign fasciculations")

5. ✓ Recurrent flu-like illness, often with chronic sore throat

6. ✓ Painful lymph nodes, especially on sides of neck and under the arms

7. ✓ Severe nasal and other allergies, often worsening of previous mild problem

8. ✓ Weight change, usually gain

9. ✓ Muscle and joint aches with tender "trigger points" or fibromyalgia

10. ✓ Abdominal pain, diarrhea, nausea, intestinal gas, "irritable bowel syndrome"

11. ✓ Low grade fevers or feeling hot often

12. ✓ Night sweats

13. ✓ Heart palpitations

14. ____ Severe premenstrual syndrome (PMS)

15. ____ Rash of herpes simplex or shingles

16. ____ Uncomfortable or recurrent urination - pain in prostate

17. ____ Other symptoms

    ____ a. rashes

    ____ b. hair loss

    ____ c. impotence

    ____ d. chest pain

_____ e. dry eyes and mouth

_____ f. cough

__✓__ g. temporomandibular joint (TMJ) syndrome

_____ h. endometriosis

_____ i. frequent canker sores

__✓__ j. cold hands and feet

_____ k. serious rhythm disturbances of the heart

_____ l. carpal tunnel syndrome

__✓__ m. pyriform muscle syndrome causing sciatica

_____ n. thyroid inflammation

__✓__ o. various cancers

_____ p. periodontal (gum) disease

_____ q. mitral valve prolapse

__✓__ r. easily getting out of breath ("dyspnea or exertion")

__✓__ s. symptoms worsened by extremes of temperature

__✓__ t. multiple sensitivities to medicine, food, and other substances

— rapid wt gain

Additional comments: Talwin alleviates fatigue, improves mood, concentration & energy. / I feel hyper & agitated most of the time even though I have no energy. / When I get over-tired & can't rest I "space out" & become very irritable & almost start crying from the exhaustion. / Slurred speech / Very poor coordination — nausea

During Lyme Disease, had visual hallucinations —

Gabapentin — mood elevation — energizing ? dizzying

The idea that CFS is a cytokine-mediated disorder was strengthened by frequent detection of various T-lymphocyte markers suggesting immune activation. Cytokines are produced when T-lymphocytes are activated. In 1987 and 1988 I found that HLA-DR and IL-2 receptor levels were increased in some patients, and that many had an increased CD4/CD8 ratio, perhaps indicating inadequate suppression of the immune response, although a subset of CD8 cells measuring numbers of cytotoxic T-lymphocytes was frequently elevated. Beta-2 microglobulin, a measure of T-cell receptor turnover, was virtually never increased. I was not able to measure serum neopterin at the time, but other workers have recently reported it to be sometimes elevated.[16] Dr. Cheney finds the soluble CD8 receptor to be elevated in about 50% of patients. He states that IL-2R and CD8R levels can be used as measures of disease activity in CFS, perhaps being the elusive "CFS sed rate" many of us have been looking for.

In an attempt to elucidate the genetic basis of CFS, I did HLA typing on over 100 CFS patients, with the aid of Paul Terasaki. We found that HLA-DR4 was increased (p=0.02) in this population, although not enough to use this lab test diagnostically. Our next step is to see whether those who were HLA-DR4+ differed clinically from those who were not.

A defect in natural killer (NK) cell activity is frequently seen in CFS patients. Some researchers believe this is one of the primary deficits, since NK cells are much involved in killing cells infected with herpesviruses. A frequent concomitant of CFS is reactivation of latent herpesvirus infections, and there is often an elevation in herpesvirus antibodies, perhaps due to infection, to a "super-antigen," or to inadequate suppression of B-lymphocytes manufacturing herpesvirus antibodies. A characteristic of human retroviral infections is that resistance to other microbial infections is reduced and this may be one reason why other agents, such as HHV-6, may be frequently isolated. The gene products of multiple infectious agents may need to synergize to produce the characteristic syndrome. It may be significant that HHV-6 may selectively impair NK function, although NK function is also altered by cortical lesions.[17]

None of these virologic or immunologic findings is diagnostic of CFS by itself. A minority of patients do not have any of these abnormalities. They cannot be distinguished from those who do by any clinical criteria I have used. Although I may regret writing this, at the current stage of my thinking, I believe that although these values may be useful in a comprehensive diagnostic array, they may almost be epiphenomena, and CFS must be viewed as a *psychoneuroimmunologic* disorder. The immune system cannot be dealt with in an isolated manner. It would be of great interest if CFS could be cured or successfully treated with an antiviral drug, and I certainly do not dismiss this possibility. Experimental therapies are being tested. It would be quite exciting to be able to treat "depression," of which some still think CFS is a manifestation, with antiviral chemotherapy. It may not be just a coincidence that "treatment-resistant depression" has been encountered more frequently in the last few years. There is, in my judgment, a likelihood that new strategies will be developed to treat mood disorders, for reasons I shall discuss in subsequent chapters. Although not effective in all patients, immunomodulatory therapy with H-2 blockers, gamma globulin, and Ampligen produces rather profound improvement in mood and fatigue often rapidly, and various psychoactive drugs, particularly antidepressants, cause clinical improvement as well as amelioration of various immunologic parameters. Nevertheless, I am not able to understand CFS unless it is in a psychoneuroimmunologic context, and I am not able to understand the generation of symptoms unless a part of the brain called the *limbic system* is involved. Before I discuss the evidence for CFS being a limbic encephalopathy in a dysregulated psychoneuroimmunologic network, I would like to explore some basic concepts of psychoneuroimmunology (PNI) and the structure and function of the limbic system.

REFERENCES

1. Goldstein JA. Therapeutic lessons from a family practitioner. *Therapaeia* September 23, 1981, 73-84.

2. Goldstein JA. Cimetidine in mononeucleosis. *Ann Int Med* 99(3): 410-411, 1983.

3. Linden DJ, Connor JA. Participation of postsynaptic PKC in cerebellar long-term depression in culture. *Science* 254:1656-1659, 1991.

4. Goldstein JA. Cimetidine, ranitidine, and Epstein-Barr virus infection. *Ann Intern Med* 105(1): 139,1986.

Jay A. Goldstein   13

5. Sharma HS, Nyberg F, Cervos-Navarro J, Day PK. Histamine modulates heat stress-induced changes in blood-brain barrier permeability, cerebral blood flow, brain oedema and serotonin levels: an experimental study in conscious young rats. *Neuroscience* 50(2):445-454, 1992.

6. Yunus MB. Personal communication, 1992.

7. Alvarez EO, Banzan AM. The rate of histamine in the anterior hypothalamus and its functional interaction with the hippocampus on exploratory behavior in adult male rats. *Behav Brain Res* 48:127-133, 1992.

8. Goldstein JA. Presented at: The First Annual Meeting of the National CEBV Syndrome Association. Portland, OR, November 4-7, 1987.

9. Goldstein JA. Presented at: First Annual Governor's Conference on Chronic Fatigue Syndrome. Newport, RI, October 1988.

10. Goldstein JA. *Chronic Fatigue Syndrome: The Struggle for Health*. Los Angeles: Chronic Fatigue Syndrome Institute, 1990.

11. Blalock JE and Smith EM. A complete regulatory loop between the immune and neuroendocrine systems. Fed Proc, FASEB 44:108-111,1985.

12. Pert CV, Ruff MR, Weber RJ, Herkenham M. Neuropeptides and their receptors: a psychosomatic network. *J Immunol* 132(2 Suppl): 1805-1826, 1985.

13. Hyde B. A historical review of M.E./CFS-like disease. In: *The Clinical and Scientific Basis of Myalgic Encephalomyelitis/Chronic Fatigue Syndrome*. Ottawa: The Nightingale Research Foundation, 1992.

14. Wessely S. History of postviral fatigue syndrome. *Br Med Bull* 47(4): 919-941, 1991.

15. Gallo R. *Virus Hunting, AIDS, Cancer, and the Human Retrovirus: A Story of Scientific Discovery*. New York, Basic Books, 1991.

16. Chao CC, Janoff EN, Hu S, Thomas K, Gallagher M, Tsong M, Peterson PK. Altered cytokine release in peripheral blood mononuclear cell cultures from patients with the chronic fatigue syndrome. Cytokine 3(4): 292-298, 1991.

17. Renoux G, Renoux M. Imuthiol, a specific immunopotentiator. *Int J Immunotherapy* VI(1): 25-35,1990.

What Is Psychoneuroimmunology (PN

SUMMARY. The historical attempts at relating "state of mind" to bodily dysfunction are reviewed. The study of stress and its role in inducing somatic dysfunction marked the first widely accepted model of psychoneuroimmunology (PNI). The "body in stress" involves, among other consequences, increased activity of the hypothalamic-pituitary-adrenal (HPA) axis and a resultant rise in glucocorticoid secretion. Other reactions to stress can involve thymic hormones and interleukin-1 (IL-1). Under certain conditions lymphocytes and macrophages can also secrete CRH and ACTH and other neuropeptide substances. This process involves "cross talk" between the central nervous system and the immune system, involving "bi-directional" networks. Viral diseases can cause neuropsychological deficits, and this process has been well documented. HIV is one example of an infectious virus inducing a neurological dementia. The response of the immune system to virally-induced stress may be genetically determined and could explain why not everyone gets chronic fatigue syndrome when exposed to the same infectious agents. Thus PNI is an important aspect of chronic fatigue syndrome, as is the role of the limbic system in regulatory physiology.

Since the initial description of CFS, and even before, in the days of epidemics of myalgic encephalomyelitis (ME) in Britain, there has been little understanding of how the symptoms of the illness could be generated. From my experience with CFS researchers and

[DocuSerial™ co-indexing entry]

"What Is Psychoneuroimmunology (PNI)?" Goldstein, J.A. Published in: *Haworth Library of the Medical Neurobiology of Somatic Disorders* (The Haworth Medical Press), Volume 1, 1993 and *Chronic Fatigue Syndromes: The Limbic Hypothesis*, Goldstein, J.A., The Haworth Medical Press, 1993.

commentators over the past six years, it has become apparent to me that those studying the illness, although well-intentioned, were products of their specialty training–usually in virology, immunology, hematology, or infectious diseases. Those who may have been properly trained, the psychoneuroimmunologists, were few in number, and were either uninformed about the disorder or did not have clinical experience dealing with patients.

There is a long tradition in medicine of the effect of mental state on immune function. Numerous commentaries about stress and bereavement, as well as psychiatric illness, discuss compromising immune function. A report of phagocytic activity of tubercle bacilli being decreased during periods of emotional stress was published by William Osler in 1919. This promising start was not as productively followed up in the United States as it might have been, perhaps due to the influence of psychoanalysis on the study of brain and behavior. The misguided theorizing of the Franz Alexander school about the psychodynamic background of organ choice for illness had an enormous impact on psychosomatic medicine in the 1950s and 1960s, and retarded investigation into the physiologic basis of neuroimmune regulation. Since biological psychiatry or behavioral neurology was virtually unknown in medical curricula at the time, psychoanalytic theory was all that many young physicians were presented with. Psychoactive drugs were in use then, but no one knew very much about how they worked. I never read anything about the interaction between the brain and the immune system that used the scientific method until I was in private practice. Even today, suggestions that the central nervous system is directly involved in causing the symptoms of CFS and related disorders are not well accepted, although many, if not most, of the symptoms are obviously neurologic. Too many of those investigating the immunology of CFS view the immune system as isolated and self-regulating. This view has become untenable in immunology in the last few years or so, but it was a common experience for me during the late 1980s to speak to researchers about cognitive dysfunction in their patients and to hear that this aspect of the illness had not been considered. The tendency of a scientist to fit patients into the Procrustean bed of his specialty interest is quite marked in chronic fatigue syndrome.

There is some agreement that there is immune dysfunction in CFS, although, as is the case with depression, most commentators are unsure about what the dysfunction is. Many immune studies have been performed, but all patients will not have a single repeatable abnormality, and some will not have any. This state of affairs represents the heterogeneity of response to specific immune stimuli among individuals, and perhaps indicates that there is more than one kind of immune stimulus involved in producing CFS, or that the immune disorders are secondary to a primary neurologic process.

The way that stress could influence human behavior was described in the pioneering work of Hans Selye in the mid-1950s, and in the stress scales of Holmes and Rahe in the mid-1960s. The study of stress responses was one of the earliest "reputable" scientific endeavors relating to PNI, since it was generally accepted that stress could influence susceptibility to several illnesses. However, it was not until the more recent demonstration that soluble immune mediators could gain access to the CNS and possibly affect the course of an illness, did PNI seriously attract attention. The process of elucidation of how psychological factors and physical stress alter the functioning of the individual is still going on, but the trickle of publications has turned into a flood.

Stress may be defined as the reaction of the body to stimuli which disturb homeostasis. The stress response has generally been assumed to involve increased activity of the hypothalamic-pituitary-adrenal (HPA) axis with a resultant rise in glucocorticoid secretion. The adrenal medulla is also stimulated, producing a release of catecholamines. Although these concepts are central in PNI, they may not apply to CFS, as we shall see in later chapters. CFS stress responses may be characterized by a decreased HPA activity, perhaps due to hyposecretion of corticotropin releasing hormone (CRH), with a decreased production of catecholamines as well. Decreased CRH levels in the CNS may account for some CFS symptoms. IL-1 alpha and/or beta may be increased in the periphery of CNS, but do not produce the expected rise in CRH and ACTH (adrenocorticotrophic hormone).

Because of stress research and the general state of scientific knowledge and technology, early work in PNI was largely neuroendocrine in orientation, and the role of the HPA axis is probably the best studied area. ACTH secretion is regulated by hypothalamic CRH, vasopressin, and oxytocin. CRH secretion is controlled by monoamines, acetylcholine, IL-1 beta, PGF_2 alpha, IL-6, and possibly protein kinases C and A.

Importantly for PNI, ACTH and CRH secretion can also be regulated by the thymic hormones and interleukin-1 (IL-1), which is secreted during various stressful situations, both outside the CNS and within it. Under certain conditions, lymphocytes and macrophages can secrete CRH and ACTH as well as numerous other neuropeptide substances. It is not known precisely what effect these agents have on physiology in health and disease when secreted by immunocytes. An important principle of PNI is that immunocytes serve as mobile sensory organs for the CNS, manufacturing local and systemic neuropeptide and immunologic transmitters when suitably stimulated. They inform the brain about local invaders and altered self-antigens and mobilize the neuroendocrine system to defend against them. The list of them is long, and growing all the time. It includes somatostatin, proopiomelanocortin and its breakdown products, vasoactive intestinal peptide (VIP), thyroid stimulating hormone (TSH), human chorionic gonadotropin (HCG), follicle stimulating hormone (FSH), luteinizing hormone (LH), and calcitonin-gene-related peptide (CGRP). The neurotransmitters and hormones that have immunomodulatory properties include those just mentioned, plus glucocorticoids, catecholamines, thyroxine, acetylcholine, sex hormones, vasopressin, oxytocin, and melatonin. There is, therefore, a great opportunity for "cross-talk" between the immune and neuroendocrine systems which may be involved in disease processes.

There are receptors on the cells of the immune system for all of the above substances, allowing for the so-called "bidirectional communication" between the immune and neuroendocrine systems, one of the basic tenets of PNI. A corollary of this finding may be that immune function is not just regulated intrinsically by the idiotypic-antiidiotypic networks first described by Jerne[1] but may also involve immunocyte-derived neuroendocrine hormones. The receptors for neuropeptides on immunocytes and hormonal cells may be products of the same gene, an interesting possibility which demonstrates the integration of the immune and neuroendocrine systems. Patients with major depression were given a thyrotropin releasing hormone (TRH) test and were found to have a blunted TSH response.[2] Stimulated lymphocytes from these patients did not produce TSH in response to TRH although those of normal patients did. Measuring receptors on lymphocytes is a good index of neuronal receptor number and type, except for alpha-adrenergic receptors, which are poorly expressed on lymphocytes. They are present on platelets, however, where they are increased in fibromyalgic patients with Raynaud's disorder.[3]

Besides the work of Blalock and Pert mentioned in the introduction, that of Hugh Besedovsky and his associates is important in understanding bidirectional communication.[4] He also views the immune system as being a "receptor sensorial organ" and has demonstrated that the hypothalamus and the limbic system respond to activation of the immune system as they would to other types of "somatic" receptors. Characteristic endocrine and autonomic changes were demonstrated to occur, and increases in nerve activity in specific hypothalamic and limbic areas were also found. His group also showed that IL-1 can stimulate ACTH and hence glucocorticoid synthesis. IL-1 was thought to be the most likely mediator of glucocorticoid changes induced by certain viruses. IL-1 can also decrease thyroid gland function, increase slow-wave sleep, and produce fever. In line with the concept of the immune system's being a receptor sensorial organ that responds to alterations in an internal self-image, Besedovsky and del Rey postulate a "code based on combinations of soluble messengers which could inform the central nervous system about the type of immune response in operation." The brain can also be informed about the location of the immune response since there is direct neural innervation of lymphoid organs and even individual immunocytes. The response of the organism will therefore be determined by the immune and neuroendocrine systems acting in a network. The implications of this important concept will be further explored in later chapters.

CFS may be caused by a virus, at least in certain patients. A viral infection perturbs the network. One might ask how the organism perceives the difference between the code elicited by the stress of a viral infection (particularly if the virus also infects the brain but primarily alters function and not structure) and that of a psychogenic stress. These are also topics that will be considered.

The notion that viral diseases could cause neuropsychological deficits is not new. The influenza epidemic of 1918 produced encephalitis lethargica and suggested that viral agents could cause psychosis. In recent years, HIV infection has sometimes been noted to present with dementia or psychiatric disturbances as the initial manifestation of the illness. Temporal lobe epilepsy is thought to be virally induced at times, and there is a growing psychiatric literature about the possible viral etiology of many syndromes.[5] Mice neonatally infected with HIV-1 are hyperactive.[6] The behavioral alterations are thought to be produced by viral antigen and inflammation in the brain, especially by altering cerebellar granule cell migration, as well as being affected by congenital resistance of the immune system. Neonatally infected mice do not develop cerebellar lesions after infection with Tamiami virus, for example.

The response of the immune system to virally induced stress is genetically determined, and it seems possible that susceptibility to viral encephalitis might be genetically determined, in part, by expression of receptors that may also provide portals of entry for viruses. Such receptor expression, particularly in the limbic system, could also be influenced by toxic factors, other viruses, immune status alteration, physical stress, and psychosocial factors. This concept would explain why not everyone gets CFS (if there is a viral etiology) and why patients develop it at certain times. It is possible that those genetically predisposed to develop affective disorders may also make cell surface receptors for "Agent X" on immunocytes and neural cells to a greater extent than those who are unaffected, assuming that "Agent X" is a retrovirus.

Neuroendocrine dysfunction affecting the hormonal substances involved in immunoregulation has now been demonstrated in CFS.[7] CRH tests are mildly abnormal, and ACTH stimulation tests sometimes show decreased cortisol production. Twenty-four hour urinary free cortisol is often borderline low. This result may be due to central hyposecretion of CRH. Prolactin levels are occasionally elevated in the absence of pituitary adenomas. Administration of bromocriptine, which could lower prolactin secretion, or a neuroleptic, which would raise it, has no effect on CFS. Polycystic ovarian disease is fairly common, suggesting a defect in LH and FSH. HCG administration has no benefit in CFS. Sleep disorders and circadian rhythm disturbances are very common, although melatonin levels have not been determined. CFS patients are very susceptible to sleep cycle disruptions such as shift change or jet lag. Thyroid autoantibodies are frequently seen, and results of systematic TRH testing have been published in fibromyalgia, demonstrating a blunted response.[8] Growth hormone stimulation tests have not been performed in CFS patients to my knowledge, but somatomedin-C/insulin-like growth factor 1 levels are decreased in fibromyalgia.[9] Analgesia is sometimes seen with administration of somatostatin octreotide (Sandostatin), which mimics the action of somatostatin and would block the effects of VIP and substance P.[10] The results are not impressive enough to implicate any of these three hormones in the pathophysiology of the illness. Hormonal modulation has only limited effects in treating CFS, as we shall see when discussing PMS and irritable bowel syndrome (IBS).

Now that aspects of PNI relevant to CFS have been discussed, let us turn to a description of the physiology of the limbic system, the part of the brain most responsible for the generation of the symptoms of CFS.

REFERENCES

1. Jerne NK. Towards a network theory of the immune system. *Annales d'Immunologie (Paris)* 125C:373-389, 1974.

2. Loosen PT. The TRH-induced TSH response in psychiatric patients: A possible neuroendocrine marker. *Psychoneuroendocrinology* 10:237-260, 1985.

3. Bennett RM, Clark SR, Campbell O, Ingram SB, Burckhardt CS, Nelson DL, Porter JM. Symptoms of Raynaud's syndrome in patients with fibromyalgia: a study using the Nielsen test, digital photoplethysmography, and measurements of platelet alpha-2 adrenegic receptors. *Arth and Rheum* 34(3): 264-269, 1991.

4. Besedovsky HO, and del Rey A. Physiological implications of the immune-neuro-endocrine network. In: Ader R, Felten DF, and Cohen N, (eds.). *Psychoneuroimmunology*, second edition, San Diego, Academic Press, 1991.

5. Kurstak E, (ed.). *Psychiatry and Biological Factors*. New York: Plenum Medical, 1991.

6. Crnic LS. Behavioral consequences of virus infection. In: Ader R, Felten DF, and Cohen N (eds.). *Psychoneuroimmunology*, second edition. San Diego: Academic Press, 1991.

7. Demitrack MA, Dale JK, Straus SE, Love L, Listwak SL, Kruesi MJP, Chrousos GP, Gold PW. Evidence for impaired activation of the hypothalamic-pituitary-adrenal axis in patients with chronic fatigue syndrome. *J Clin Endocrinol Metab* 73(6): 1224-1234, 1991.

8. Neeck G, Riedel W. Thyroid function in patients with fibromyalgia syndrome. *J Rheumatol* 19:1120-1122, 1992.

9. Bennett RM, Clark SR, Campbell SM, Burckhardt CS. Low somatomedin-C levels in fibromyalgia (poster). Presented at American College of Rheumatology, 55th annual scientific meeting, November 17-21, 1991, Boston.

10. Wolfe F, Mullins M, Cathey MS. A double blind placebo controlled trial of somatostatin in fibromyalgia (poster). Presented at American College of Rheumatology, 55th Annual Scientific Meeting, November 17-21, 1991, Boston.

The Limbic System

SUMMARY. The major structures of the limbic system in the brain, the hippocampus and the amygdala, are reviewed. The interaction of the various structures that comprise the limbic system is discussed. The limbic system is considered to be a neural network which can be mapped with monoclonal antibodies. Certain viral infections, such as Borna virus, have a predilection for the limbic system. Other limbic attributes are receptors for biogenic amines and neuropeptides, afferent and efferent neurons, and modulation by endogenous opioids, as well as interleukin-1, which has effects on slow-wave sleep, appetite, and fever. Mood and memory disorders have traditionally been associated with the limbic system, but recent discoveries in neurophysiology suggest that limbic dysregulation can produce illness behavior as well as dysfunction in many organ systems. Cells that secrete dopamine, norepinephrine, and serotonin are distributed throughout the brain stem and project to the limbic system. Limbic physiology is described as "medicine's stepchild," and disorders related to it have generally been labeled "psychiatric," and not part of hard medical science. The concept of the limbic system as a neural regulator is a new one, but limbic dysfunction may produce the symptoms of chronic fatigue syndrome.

I have come to the conclusion that most of the symptoms of CFS can be explained by postulating a limbic encephalopathy. Although the data to support this belief have an experimental grounding, it would still be a rational assertion if one just applies the contempo-

---

[DocuSerial™ co-indexing entry]

"The Limbic System," Goldstein, J.A. Published in: *Haworth Library of the Medical Neurobiology of Somatic Disorders* (The Haworth Medical Press), Volume 1, 1993 and *Chronic Fatigue Syndromes: The Limbic Hypothesis,* Goldstein, J.A., The Haworth Medical Press, Inc., 1993.

23

rary concept of limbic system anatomy and physiology to explain how the symptoms complex of CFS could be generated. But first, a discussion of what the limbic system is and how it works is in order.

Most physicians I have spoken with have only the vaguest notion of the limbic system. They may recall that it was mentioned in medical school lectures on neuroanatomy in reference to emotion, and some may remember the "Papez circuit," a reverberating system for the generation of emotions described in 1937. A few researchers in behavioral neurology and physiological psychology may regard a discussion of the limbic system as "gratuitous" (as one of them termed it), but a leading specialist in CFS recently asked me, "What's in the limbic system?" I expect that in the next few years a detailed knowledge of the workings of the limbic system will be necessary to understand many presently mysterious medical disorders. For the present, a general discussion should suffice.

The major structures of the limbic system are the hippocampus and the amygdala. Both are located in the medial part of the anterior temporal lobe, a region which is quite sensitive to anoxic damage and viral infection, notably by HSV-1. It is well accepted that the hippocampus is involved in the making of new memories, a process called "encoding." Although the hippocampus has several input (afferent) systems, it has only one major output (efferent) system: the fornix. This structure, also part of the limbic system, terminates in the mammillary bodies, part of the hypothalamus. Thus the hippocampus can have a significant neuroendocrine-autonomic function as well as its better known roles in memory and emotion. It is divided into four areas (CA1-4) on the basis of histological and functional criteria. The CA1 section is the most sensitive to hypoxic insult.

The amygdala is another structure involved in memory and emotion, although its role in the generation of affect has been accorded more prominence. In contradistinction to the hippocampus, the amygdala has a large number of afferents and efferents. Its various nuclei communicate with hypothalamic, thalamic, striatal, cortical, and brain stem structures, and are directly involved in the regulation of many (if not most) of the homeostatic functions in man.

In lower mammals, the olfactory lobes and piriform cortex are a major input to the limbic system. Although these pathways still exist in man, they have been superseded by visual pathways, particularly those from the orbitofrontal cortex in the inferior portion of the frontal lobe. This part of the cortex is included in the limbic system, and, along with the insula and cingulate cortex, has direct pathways to the brain stem, particularly to structures in the midbrain and pons. A contemporary description of the components of the limbic system would include the hippocampus, amygdala, piriform cortex, septal nuclei, cingulate gyrus, anterior insula, orbitofrontal cortex, nonspecific thalamic nuclei, hypothalamus (especially the anterior portion), "limbic striatum" (including the nucleus accumbens and mesolimbic dopaminergic tracts), and the midbrain tegmental area.

For practical purposes, one can consider most of the components of the limbic system as being interconnected, although this dictum is not strictly true. The limbic system is a neuronal network; some of the connections are not obvious, or may be inferred. As one neurology professor remarked to me when I asked him about possible limbic connections to the cerebellum (admitting that he had never been good at neuroanatomy): "Everything is connected to everything else."

The limbic system is now considered to be a functional unit, but it can also be mapped with monoclonal antibodies, indicating that there is an antigenic commonality among these various structures. Certain viral infections have a predilection for the limbic system as a whole, Borna virus being the best known. There are also paraneoplastic syndromes such as "limbic encephalitis" which are characterized by limbic inflammation, thought to occur on an autoimmune or viral basis.

The limbic system has receptors for monoamines. There is a high density of serotonin receptors in the amygdala and hippocampus. One type of serotonin receptor, the 5HT-1C receptor, is found primarily in the hippocampus and choroid plexus.[1] When specific ligands for this receptor are developed (current agents crossreact with the 5HT-2 receptor), pharmacologic probing of limbic function will be more precise. Although the limbic system has receptors for virtually all neuropeptides, those of particular interest are enkephalin and CRH receptors. The limbic system is particularly rich in afferents and efferents of these neurons. Endogenous opioids have a number of well-known interactions with other transmitter substances, but one which has recently been appreciated is that with interleukin-1 (IL-1).

IL-1 has been known for some time to have effects on the brain. Its roles in induction of slow-wave sleep, appetite, and fever production are well recognized. Although made peripherally and unable to cross the blood-brain barrier, it can have effects on the brain through the circumventricular organs (CVO) which allow some penetration of peripheral substances that cannot enter elsewhere. It has been proposed that IL-1 beta rarely enters the brain via the CVOs, but rather, a message is transduced to CVO neurons to manufacture the same cytokines and neuropeptides as are present in the peripheral circulation that contacts the CVOs.[2]

IL-1 is manufactured in the brain and so are its receptors. The areas of highest activity by far are the granule cells of the dentate gyrus of the hippocampus and the choroid plexus.[3] The effect of IL-1 as a neurotransmitter may be mediated, at least in part, by endogenous opioid peptides.[4] IL-1 can suppress an LH surge by inhibiting the release of leutinizing hormone releasing hormone (LHRH). This inhibition can be blocked by naloxone. IL-1 and IL-6 stimulate the release of corticotropin releasing hormone from rat hypothalamus in vitro via the eicosanoid cyclooxygenase pathway, so the effects of IL-1 in the brain are not exclusively mediated by opioids.[5] The role of hippocampal secretion of IL-1 is presently speculative. IL-1 beta has been found to inhibit long-term potentiation in the CA3 region of mouse hippocampal slices.[6] The CNS localization of other cytokines has not been well described at the time of this writing. A cytokine excess hypothesis does not mesh with a CRH deficiency state, but interference with central cytokine function could explain the situation.

The anatomy and physiology of the limbic system is very complex and it is not my intention to cover it here in detail. Interested readers are referred to standard neuroanatomy texts as well as to *The Limbic System: Functional Organization and Clinical Disorders,* edited by B.K. Doane and K.F. Livingston, New York, Raven Press, 1986. A detailed description of the functional neuroanatomy of the limbic system, as well as thought-provoking evolutionary speculation of its structures, may be found in *The Triune Brain in*

Evolution: Role in Paleocerebral Functions, by Paul D. MacLean, New York, Plenum Press, 1990. Interested readers are also referred to *The Amygdala: Neurobiological Aspects of Emotion, Memory, and Mental Dysfunction,* edited by John P. Aggleton, New York, Wiley-Liss, 1992. This book provides a unique description of the extraordinarily complex neuroanatomic and neurochemical mechanisms of this integral component of the limbic system and gives one an appreciation of the multitude of pathways that modulate limbic physiology.

For the purposes of this discussion it is most important to have an understanding of the regulatory function of the limbic system, or the "visceral brain" as it has been termed by Paul MacLean. The limbic system acts as a buffer between the internal and external world. Its efferents are to highly specialized areas of the cerebral cortex, and also to the instinctual parts of the nervous system in the lower brain stem, spinal cord, and autonomic nervous system. MacLean assigns a specific priority to the hippocampus in this regard: "Since the hippocampal formation receives connections from all the limbic areas innervated by extero- and interoceptive systems, it is in a position to achieve a synthesis of internally and externally derived information, and, in turn, to influence the activity of the hypothalamus and other structures involved in somatovisceral functions variously called upon in self-preservation, procreation, and family-related behavior."[7] Chronic fatigue syndrome may be viewed as a dysregulation of a hippocampal neural network. The temporal lobe limbic system exerts its functional role primarily by projecting directly to the diencephalon, midbrain, and spinal cord, according to Poletti.[8]

It is not well known by most physicians that the frontal lobe is the highest level of integration of autonomic function. Lesions or stimulation of this area can cause changes in bowel and bladder control as well as in temperature and sweating. Other cortical areas are involved in autonomic regulation as well. These cortical areas–the insula, and portions of the temporal and parietal lobes–are generally included in the limbic system.

Nevertheless, the role of the limbic system has traditionally been concerned with emotion and memory, and with any effects on other bodily functions considered to be associated with emotional reactions essential to survival of the species. The notion that the limbic system is a high order regulatory structure in the neuroendocrine immune network that may be involved in consciousness and the interface of mind and body does not seem to be adequately appreciated by many researchers and has certainly not filtered down to the level of the practicing physician.

The neuroscientist who has most influenced me in the development of my thinking about the limbic system is M-Marsel Mesulam, MD, whose book, *Principles of Behavioral Neurology,* Philadelphia: F.A. Davis, 1985, I heartily recommend. Much of the rest of this chapter will draw on his work. Other works of interest include:

1. Reynolds EH, Trimble MR. *The Bridge Between Neurology and Psychiatry.* Edinburgh, Churchill Livingstone, 1989.
2. Joseph R. *Neurology, Neuropsychiatry and Behavioral Neurology.* New York, Plenum Press, 1990.
3. Fuster JM. *The Prefrontal Cortex: Anatomy, Physiology and Neuropsychology of the Frontal Lobe,* 2nd edition. New York, Raven Press, 1989.
4. Lishman WA. *Organic Psychiatry: The Psychological Consequences of Cerebral Disorder,* 2nd edition. Oxford, Blackwell, 1987.

LIMBIC SYSTEM PHYSIOLOGY

The cerebral cortex may be divided on the basis of structure, from simple and undifferentiated ("corticoid") to complex. The amygdaloid nuclei and septal nuclei are examples of corticoid structures. "Allocortical" structures have one or two layers of neurons. The hippocampus and piriform cortex are allocortical structures. The corticoid and allocortical structures comprise the basic limbic system.

Areas around the limbic system are called "paralimbic" and have a more complex "meso-cortical" histologic structure. There are five major paralimbic structures in man:

1. The caudal orbitofrontal cortex
2. The insula

3. The temporal pole
4. The parahippocampal gyrus
5. The cingulate cortex

These regions form a ring, or "limbus" around the base of the brain.

Most of the cortical surface is composed of the homotypical association areas which can be divided into unimodal and hetero- modal types. Unimodal cortex is confined to one sensory modality, such as hearing. The heteromodal isocortex has neuronal responses that are not specific to one single sensory modality. The heteromo- dal isocortex is more similar in structure to the paralimbic cortex than is the unimodal isocortex. The idiotypic cortical regions are the well known highly differentiated, primary visual, auditory, somato- sensory, and motor cortices. Mesulam has devised a schema for understanding how this anatomical organization is related to func- tion and behavior (see Figure 1).

There are five types of cortex that range from the simplest to the most differentiated. The location in the brain of these cortical types suggests how they may be functionally related.

The limbic structures are most closely associated with the hypo- thalamus, the basic regulator of the internal milieu and generator of drives and instincts. The limbic system is involved with many of the same functions as the hypothalamus, as well as being more in- volved in memory and learning, and certain social functions unique to mammals which are important for survival of the species. The idiotypic cortex at the other pole of the schema is scarcely in- fluenced by limbic activity, since it would not serve the organism well to have primary sensory input and motor instructions colored by emotions or drive state. Unimodal association cortex processes this input in a fairly pure form, a task also vital for survival.

The heteromodal and paralimbic areas also process this informa- tion, but in a more "general" way. They integrate it into drive, affect, experience, and, if you will, "personality." The idiotypic and unimodal cortical areas are "dedicated" to one modality of information transfer, while the heteromodal-paralimbic areas have many inputs and outputs and cannot be assigned a specialization.

Mesulam's schema also addresses neuroanatomical connectivit

FIGURE 1. Cortical zones of the human brain.

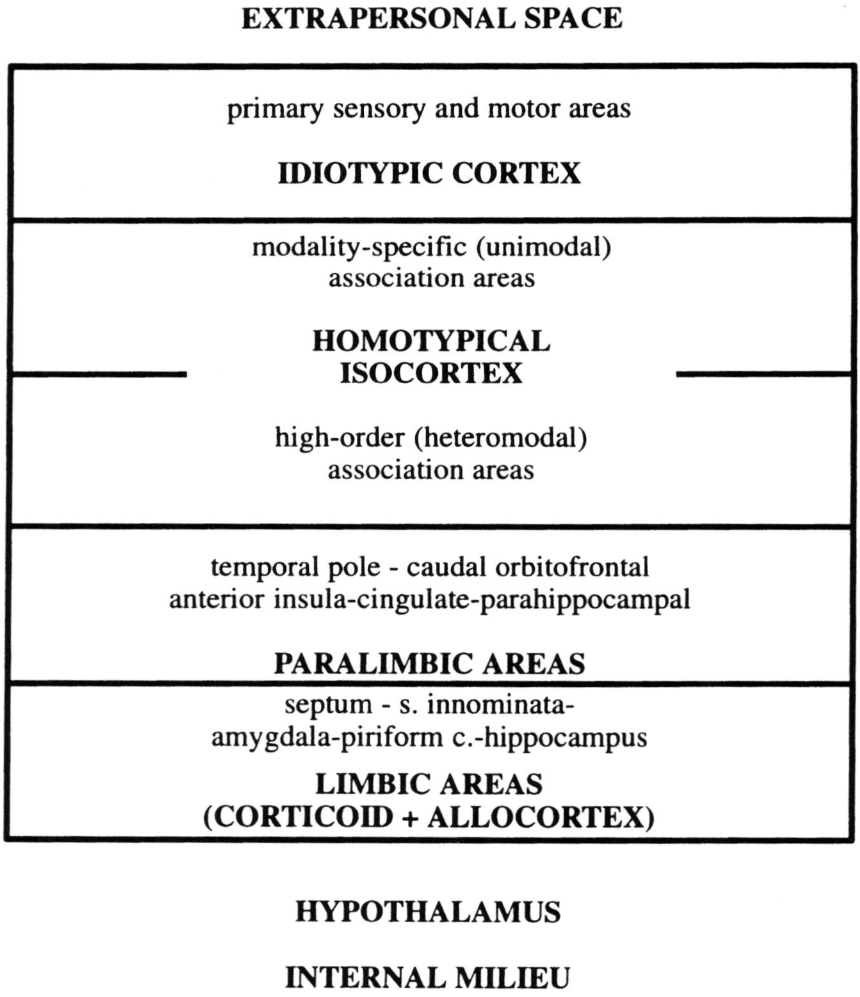

EXTRAPERSONAL SPACE

primary sensory and motor areas **IDIOTYPIC CORTEX**
modality-specific (unimodal) association areas **HOMOTYPICAL ISOCORTEX** high-order (heteromodal) association areas
temporal pole - caudal orbitofrontal anterior insula-cingulate-parahippocampal **PARALIMBIC AREAS**
septum - s. innominata- amygdala-piriform c.-hippocampus **LIMBIC AREAS (CORTICOID + ALLOCORTEX)**

HYPOTHALAMUS

INTERNAL MILIEU

Adjacent areas communicate with each other much more than do non-adjacent areas. For example, the hypothalamus and limbic system have many direct communications and influences, whereas, with few exceptions, the direct hypothalamic influences on the rest of the cortex are relatively minor.

The anatomic localization of the heteromodal areas, which can provide substantial preprocessed sensory information to the motivational areas of the paralimbic cortex, is not well known in general medicine. These areas include the prefrontal cortex, the supramarginal gyrus, the medial parieto-occipital area, the inferior parietal lobule and the angular gyrus.

The presence of heteromodal and paralimbic areas has been described as a "synaptic buffer" between external reality and internal urges. They provide the individual with many alternative ways of responding to a certain stimulus based on its context. Rather than a programmed response pattern, behavior can be altered to meet the various contingencies of internal states, the external world, and previous experience. It is in these areas that the mind-body dilemma has its primary focus and possible solution, as genetic traits and neural states admix to determine behavior. The distinction between "physical" and "mental" blurs so much that it becomes almost meaningless.

A discussion of the mind-body problem is certainly germane to an understanding of CFS, but the concepts involved are often abtruse and occupy a no-man's land between philosophy, cognitive neuroscience, and molecular neurobiology.

The reader is referred to the following books that consider this issue from various neurobiologic and philosophical perspectives:

- Edelman GM. *Bright Air, Brilliant Fire: On the Matter of the Mind.* New York, Basic Books, 1992.
- Carpenter GA, Grossberg S (eds.). *Pattern Recognition in Self-Organizing Neural Networks.* Cambridge, MA; MIT Press, 1991.
- Brown JW. *Self and Processs: Brain States and the Conscious Present.* New York; Springer-Verlag, 1991.

- Black IB. *Information in the Brain: A Molecular Perspective.* Cambridge, MA; MIT Press, 1991.
- Dennet D. *Consciousness Explained.* Boston; Little, Brown, 1991.

Some of these works have been reviewed in the *New England Journal of Medicine* 327 (13):1335-1339, 1992.

The involvement of the limbic system in memory is well known. An amnestic state cannot exist without limbic dysfunction. Hippocampal lesions characteristically produce impairment in the making of new memories, and when both hippocampus and amygdala are involved, the memory impairment is very severe. Since paralimbic areas transmit information from cortical sensory areas to the hippocampus, paralimbic lesions can also cause a memory impairment.

It is also accepted that paralimbic areas, along with other limbic structures, regulate drive and affect. What is not as well understood is the degree to which they determine higher autonomic control by functioning as a neuroendocrine transduction mechanism. The limbic system has traditionally been associated with emotion. Autonomic changes that occur with emotional state have been discussed in the literature, but do not seem to have been fully integrated into the functioning of the organism. The role of the amygdala in producing visceral changes has been known for many years, and more recent discoveries that electrical stimulation of paralimbic areas produces consistent changes in sleep states, gastrointestinal motility, cardiac rate, and blood pressure are helpful in our understanding of physiology and disease. Could dysfunction of the orbitofrontal cortex cause slow-wave sleep disorders and cardiac arrhythmias? Could dysfunction of the insular cortex cause irritable bowel syndrome? Since paralimbic areas are primary determinants of mental state, as discussed previously, they provide a "bridge" between anatomy and psychosomatic disease which was first discussed by MacLean in the late 1940s but has been ignored or only paid lip-service in most contemporary writings. Using the construct of heteromodal-paralimbic-limbic-hypothalamic-brain stem connectivity, it is not difficult to conceive how a potent emotional experience such as child abuse or post-traumatic stress disorder could modify synaptic connections so that normal regulation of neuroimmune function is significantly altered. This idea is related to the concept of "behavioral kindling" proposed by Robert Post.[9] He also addresses the role of sensitization in alteration of gene expression, such as the induction of the proto-oncogene c fos and related transcription factors. These may "then affect the expression of transmitters, receptors and neuropeptides that alter responsivity in a long-lasting fashion."[10] These issues will be further addressed in subsequent chapters.

THE LIMBIC ZONE

The limbic zone of the limbic system comprises the amygdala, hippocampus, piriform cortex, septal nuclei, and substantia innominata. These regions behave similarly to the paralimbic area but since they have direct synaptic connections to the hypothalamus, lesions in the limbic zone produce more profound impairment in memory, drive, affect, neuroendocrine control, autonomic tone, and immunoregulation.

Piriform cortex. The functions of the piriform cortex are incompletely understood. The olfactory lobe provides chemical input to the brain via smell and is the only sensory modality that does not have thalamic relays. It has a high density of IL-1 receptors. Whales and dolphins, however, have a piriform cortex and are reported to have no sense of smell. An animal model of depression has been produced by olfactory bulbectomy.[11] The piriform cortex connects directly to other limbic zone structures as well as to the hypothalamus and to the paralimbic regions.

Hippocampus. Although the hippocampus receives afferents from numerous structures, its efferents are generally considered to be in the fornix, which terminates in the mammillary body. There are also direct hippocampal efferents to the amygdala and septum. Via the fornix, there are indirect projections to the medial preoptic area, the anterior hypothalamus, the lateral hypothalamic area, the ventral tegmental area, and the central gray matter of the midbrain.[12] The mammillary body has diffuse projections in the brain. Hippocampal efferents are said to reach widespread areas of the cerebral cortex and amygdala in the rhesus monkey. These fibers cross to the contralateral limbic zone through commissures, as is true for those of the amygdala and piriform cortex. Mirror images of unilateral limbic lesions have been reported in the contralateral hemisphere. Although the hippocampus has been implicated in emotion and neuro-immune-endocrine regulation, its main function is in the making of memories, and in this mode virtually its entire sensory input is paralimbic. Because of this connection, there is a distinct motivational component to learning. Anxiety may be mediated in the dorsal hippocampus through the septo-hippocampal circuit, since both diazepam and tandospirone, a 5HT-1A agonist, have anti-anxiety effects when injected into the dorsal hippocampus.[13] The hippocampus may also be involved in depression, particularly in elderly depressed patients, in whom magnetic resonance imaging (MRI) revealed significantly shortened T1 spin lattice relaxation times.[14]

Amygdala. The amygdala is unique among limbic zone structures in that it has direct connections with other cortical areas, the hypothalamus, and preganglionic autonomic regions of the brain stem. Because of this anatomical evidence, the amygdala may contribute to the final common pathway for limbic mediated somatomotor and visceromotor changes. The "amygdaloid complex" is composed of several nuclei but most projections to the brain stem autonomic neurons come from the central nucleus, the most primitive from a standpoint of comparative vertebrate zoology.

Electrical stimulation of the amygdala in awake animals produces fear responses as well as apparent sympathetic nervous system arousal. There is a suggestion that the amygdala may not be involved in normal homeostatic functions since it may not function in sleep. Other studies have found, however, that amygdaloid neurons increase their rate of firing during slow-wave sleep.

The amygdala is rich in monoamine, cholinergic, and GABAergic afferents, and a high density of benzodiazepine receptors has been reported in the basolateral nucleus of the amygdala, suggesting it as a site of anxiolytic drug action. The basolateral nucleus has a dense network of communication with the central nucleus. Most of the peptides found in the brain can be localized in amygdaloid cell bodies and terminals.[15] Since amygdaloid transmitters include hormones, monoamines, eicosanoids, peptides, excitatory amino acids (EAAs) and possibly cytokines, the opportunity for quite sophisticated coding of amygdalar input and output exists, especially since there are several different interconnected amygdalar nuclei with varying functional specializations.

Cells that produce dopamine, norepinephrine, and serotonin are distributed throughout the brain stem in designated groups. Amygdalar nerves terminate on some of these cell groups and not others. These monoamine-producing cell groups project widely throughout the CNS and also back to the limbic system. Thus there is a highly complex system for modulating amygdalar inputs and outputs which has obvious implications for homeostatic function and specific types of "psychosomatic" pathophysiology. This interactive network needs considerable further study.

Basal ganglia. The basal ganglia are well known for their involvement in motor function and the extrapyramidal system. One part of the basal ganglia, the striatum, is composed of the caudate, putamen, olfactory tubercle, and nucleus accumbens. The caudate nucleus has recently received attention for its role in obsessive-compulsive disorder and Tourette's syndrome, but these are problems not usually encountered in the CFS patient. It has been implicated in memory function and pain modulation, symptoms of obvious relevance in CFS. The striatal areas which receive limbic projections are the nucleus accumbens and the olfactory tubercle. These structures are known as the limbic striatum. They have been investigated for their role in schizophrenia and have predominantly dopaminergic innervation, but involvement of these limbic mechanisms in CFS is somewhat speculative, since dopaminergic agonists or antagonists have little effect on the illness. Dopamine precursors have more of a role in experimental preparations. The other component of the basal ganglia, the globus pallidus, also has preferential limbic affiliations. Neurons in the ventral pallidum respond to amygdaloid stimulation, perhaps mediated through the nucleus accumbens.

Thalamus. The anatomy of the thalamus is very complex. This structure functions as a relay station for sensory nerve input. The thalamic nuclei with which most physicians are familiar are the lateral basal nuclei which relay sensory information to the idiotypic cortex. Other areas in the lateral basal nuclei relay to the unimodal association cortex. Large areas, however, are relays for heteromodal, paralimbic, and limbic cortices. The function of these nuclei is not well understood. The reticular and intralaminal thalamic nuclei are relays from the reticular activating system and have diffuse cortical projections. Thalamic pain is a well-recognized neurologic entity caused by destructive lesions, often strokes, in the thalamus. This sort of pain presents with little sensory loss and is often accompanied with dysesthesias and paresthesias. A more inclusive term used to describe similar types of pain resulting from dysregulation of CNS pain pathways is "central pain."

Overview. Thus the "limbic system" comprises several structures:

1. Hypothalamus
2. Limbic cortex
3. Paralimbic cortex
4. Limbic areas of the basal ganglia
5. Limbic and paralimbic thalamic nuclei
6. Midbrain ventral tegmentum including reticular nuclei
7. Possibly the serotoninergic dorsal raphe in the midbrain, which has 70% of its terminals in the limbic cortex

Limbic areas have common membrane antigens and are particularly susceptible to epileptic and behavioral kindling. All of these components are more involved with regulating the internal milieu–memory, drive, and affect–than with the elementary sensory and motor processing about which physicians have been most educated.

Limbic physiology is medicine's stepchild. Behavioral neurologists understand it as it affects behavior, and neuroscientists learn aspects of limbic function as it relates to their area of specialization. Biological psychiatrists have a sophisticated understanding of transmitters and receptors, but usually have little knowledge of the anatomy involved, which is best understood by neurosurgeons. Neuroendocrinologists usually restrict their view to the hypothalamus and pituitary as do the psychoneuroimmunologists. Disorders related to limbic physiology have generally been called "psychiatric," which has in fact meant "we really do not understand how they work but they are not part of hard medical science." The concept of the limbic system's being a neural regulator is a rather new one, but it is exquisitely suited to explaining the symptoms of chronic fatigue syndrome.

REFERENCES

1. Azmitia EC, Whitaker-Azmitia PM. Awakening the sleeping giant: anatomy and plasticity of the brain serotoninergic system. *J Clin Psychiatry* 52(Suppl): 4-16, 1991.

2. Saper CB. Neurologic origin of fever. Presented at the Seminar in Behavioral Neuroimmunology, UCLA School of Medicine, October 20, 1992.

3. Licinio J, Wong M-L, Gold PW. Localization of interleukin-l receptor antagonist mRNA in rat brain. *Endocrinology* 129(1):562-564, 1991.

4. Fagarasan MO, Arora PK, Axelrod J. Interleukin-l potentiation of beta-endorphin secretion and the dynamics of interleukin-l internalization in pituitary cells. *Prog Neuropsychopharmacol Biol Psychiatry* 15:551-560, 1991.

5. Fisher LA. Corticotropin-releasing factor: endocrine and autonomic integration of responses to stress. *Trends Pharmacol Sci* 10:189-192,1989.

6. Katsuki HZ, Nakai B, Hirai Y, Akaji J, Kiso Y, Satoh M. Interleukin-l beta inhibits long-term potentiation in the CA3 region of mouse hippocampal slices. *Eur J Pharmacol* 1818(3): 323-326, 1990.

7. MacLean PD. *The Triune Brain in Evolution: Role in Paleocerebral Functions.* New York, Plenum Press, 1990, p. 514.

8. Poletti CE. Is the limbic system a limbic system? Studies of hippocampal efferents: their functional and clinical implications. In: *The Limbic System: Functional Organization and Clinical Disorders.* Doane BE, Livingston KE (eds.). New York Raven Press, 1986.

9. Post RM, Rubinow DR, Balenger JC. Conditioning, sensitization, and kindling: implications for the course of affective illness. In: *Neurobiology of Mood Disorders.* Eds: Post RM, Ballenger JC. Baltimore, Williams and Wilkins, 1984.

10. Post RM. Transduction of psychosocial stress into the neurobiology of recurrent affective disorder. *Am J Psychiatry* 149(8):999-1010, 1992.

11. Jesberger JA, Richardson JS. Brain output dysregulation induced by olfactory bulbectomy: an approximation for the rat of major depressive disorders in humans. *Int J Neurosci* 38:241-265, 1988.

12. MacLean PD. *The Triune Brain in Evolution: Role in Paleocerebral Functions.* New York, Plenum Press, 1990.

13. Kalkman HO, Fozard JR. 5HT receptor subtypes and their role in disease. *Curr Opinion Neurol Neurosurg* 4:560-565, 1991.

14. Krishnan PR, Doraiswany PM, Figiel GS, Hosain MM, Shah SA, Na C, Boyko OB, McDonald WM, Nemeroff CB, Ellinwood EH. Hippocampal abnormalities in depression. *J Neuropsychiatry* 3(4):387-391, 1991.

15. Henke PG, Ray A, Sullivan RM. The amygdala: emotions and gut functions. *Dig Dis Sci* 36(11):1633-1643, 1991.

Chronic Fatigue Syndrome: Limbic Encephalopathy in a Dysregulated Neuroimmune Network

SUMMARY. It is difficult to integrate the array of symptoms typical of chronic fatigue syndrome. The label "psychosomatic" is often applied to illnesses that present a wide variety of "unconnected" symptoms. The "limbic encephalopathy" model requires a paradigm shift to describe the disease. Each symptom of chronic fatigue syndrome including profound physical fatigue after exertion is explained by dysfunction of the limbic mechanisms. Results of SPECT scans, showing worsened temporal and frontal hypoperfusion after exercise, and the non-restorative, alpha-EEG sleep abnormality in CFS patients are described. Other symptoms discussed in the context of limbic dysfunction are cognitive dysfunction, "encoding" of new memories, attention and concentration difficulties, intermittent blurred vision, problems with spatial relations, dyscalculia, poor impulse control, and visual agnosia. A possible relationship to early childhood trauma or post-traumatic stress disorder is proposed. Other manifestations of limbic dysfunction include irritability, anxiety, panic disorder, bruxism, restless leg syndrome, sleep apnea, disordered sleep patterns, carpal tunnel syndrome, headache, fibromyalgia, sinusitis, tinnitus, and vertigo. Note is made of recurrent flu-like illness with sore throat, limbic control of mast cell innervation, and the role of the limbic system in irritable bowel syndrome.

[DocuSerial™ co-indexing entry]

"Chronic Fatigue Syndrome: Limbic Encephalopathy in a Dysregulated Neuroimmune Network," Goldstein, J.A. Published in: *Haworth Library of the Medical Neurobiology of Somatic Disorders* (The Haworth Medical Press), Volume 1, 1993 and *Chronic Fatigue Syndromes: The Limbic Hypothesis,* Goldstein, J.A., The Haworth Medical Press, 1993.

39

Using the contemporary methods of understanding health and disease, many physicians can make no sense whatever of the multiplicity of seemingly unrelated symptoms that comprise chronic fatigue syndrome (CFS). It is unfortunately an all too common practice that if a clinical situation does not fit into established modes of analysis, then it is not regarded as being worthy of serious consideration. Often such cases are referred to psychiatrists, being labeled "psychosomatic" or "hysterical" with no further thought having been given to how such symptoms may have been generated. If one accepts that we live in a rational universe where physical laws of cause and effect operate, even the most bizarre somatic complaints then have some organic basis. To think otherwise has caused people in the not so distant past to be labeled as witches or victims of demonic possession. A somewhat less pejorative designation is that "it's all in the mind," without giving consideration to how an immaterial mind can cause effects on a material body, a conundrum which has puzzled thinkers for centuries but may be nearing solution based on scientific discoveries alluded to in previous chapters.

Another common way of dismissing a patient's complaints is by saying, "I don't know what's wrong with you–all your tests are normal." Consideration may not be given to the possibility that the appropriate test may not have been ordered, or is not yet in existence. In order to properly characterize the abnormalities seen in CFS, different and perhaps newer tests must be performed to demonstrate pathophysiology, and a new conceptual framework for diagnosis and treatment must be sought. The alternative is consigning these patients to categories such as "neurasthenia," which, although apparently quite common, have never been adequately explained.

A new way of looking at related phenomena has been called a "paradigm shift." Examples of such shifts would be the invention of Newtonian mechanics and the development of the germ theory of infectious disease. Both of these conceptualizations led to new and better ways of understanding and managing observable events that were far-reaching. I offer for your consideration the question whether viewing CFS as a limbic encephalopathy in a dysregulated neuroimmune network may also represent a paradigm shift.

LIMBIC ETIOLOGY OF SOME CFS SYMPTOMS

Fatigue

Fatigue is obviously an important component of CFS although it may not necessarily be present in related disorders. Very little (almost nothing) of substance has been published about how fatigue is produced. What has been written generally concludes that fatigue may be produced by muscular exertion, but there is little agreement about the cause of muscle fatigue. An article by Robert Layzer in the *New England Journal of Medicine* in February of 1991[1] reached no specific conclusion, although subsequent letters to the editor suggested hyperkalemia or depletion of adenosine triphosphate (ATP). A possibly pathognomonic alteration in an anti-viral enzyme known as 2´,5´ oligoadenylate synthetase/RNase L may account for fatigue in CFS because activation of the pathway to manufacture this enzyme consumes ATP, and very high levels of the enzyme are seen in the majority of those with CFS participating in double-blind trials of the immunomodulatory agent Ampligen.[2] CFS fatigue increases with exercise but often not until several hours later. Other symptoms also may be markedly worsened by exercise.

A more compelling hypothesis is that the fatigue is inappropriately generated by the central nervous system. CFS patients commonly develop fatigue unrelated to physical exertion: they can wake up fatigued, may become fatigued from stress, odors, trauma, circadian oscillations, or from no apparent cause. Cardiopulmonary exercise and muscle testing may reveal minor abnormalities in oxygen consumption and anaerobic threshold, and magnetic resonance spectroscopy may detect fairly trivial deficiencies in ATP. None of these abnormalities would be sufficient to explain the profound, devastating fatigue that these patients feel, which is often delayed after exercise by a day or so. A common report of a patient who completed exercise testing fairly well is that he became so exhausted the next day that he had to stay in bed for up to a week. There is reason to suggest that fatigue could be qualitatively similar to other complex sensations such as hunger, pain, or sleepiness. These states are characterized by regulation in several locations in the neuraxis (and possibly elsewhere in a neural network) and are mediated by multiple transmitter substances. Occasionally a CFS patient will become manic or hypomanic and have a complete resolution of fatigue during this period. More often, however, the patient will feel energized and driven but will still fatigue very easily, perhaps more so since he is overextending himself.

The most convincing clinical experience suggesting a central cause for fatigue is that of George Karpati, a neuropathologist at the Montreal Neurological Institute, where Wilder Penfield did his pioneering neurosurgical work. Dr. Karpati reports on stereotactic brain stimulation in patients with intractable epilepsy being considered for ablative surgery. Some of the patients, when being stimulated in the medial temporal lobe, report a sudden onset of severe fatigue, "like someone turned on a faucet and drained all the energy out of me."[3] Although electrode stimulation of the brain is an imprecise technique, this finding is what one would expect. The amygdala and hippocampus are located in the medial temporal lobe, as is the dentate gyrus adjacent to the hippocampus. The granule cells of the dentate gyrus have the highest concentration of IL-1 receptors in the brain, and if cytokines are involved in causing fatigue, as one would expect from the fatiguing malaise associated with infections and therapeutic administration of alpha interferon and interleukin-2, the medial temporal lobe is where a fatigue center should be.

Almost always, the fatigue in CFS is made worse by exercise. This characteristic is one of the many which distinguish CFS from major depressive disorder (MDD). Exercise or exertion of any sort can cause the CFS patient to relapse in virtually every respect. This unusual tendency may be better understood with the knowledge that certain cytokine levels are increased by exercise. The mechanism of this increase is unclear at present, and there is no information about levels of CNS cytokines pre- and post-exercise. Marathon runners often develop flu-like symptoms after a race. IL-1, the only cytokine studied to any great extent for its effects on the brain, increases after exercise. Its effects on behavior can be explained by its uptake by, or influence on, various circumventricular organs where the blood-brain-barrier is rudimentary. Otherwise, the blood-brain barrier is impermeable to IL-1. The improvement in CFS symptoms sometimes seen with gradually increasing exercise levels could be due to a desensitization of limbic cytokine receptors. One characteristic of Ampligen responders was high serum levels of IL-1 alpha.

When [133]Xenon brain SPECT scans of the brain are performed pre- and post-exercise in CFS, the temporal and frontal hypoperfusion characteristically seen is significantly worsened.[5] This response is paradoxical, since exercise in normal people will increase regional cerebral blood flow, if it will affect it at all. The reason for this effect is unclear. The only study on the effects of cytokines on cerebral perfusion was done in rats.[6] IL-2 reduced the efficacy of cerebral vasodilator and vasoconstrictive agents, but did not alter perfusion in and of itself. Receptors for IL-1 and IL-1 receptor antagonist mRNA are dense in cerebral vasculature, but their function is poorly understood.[7] IL-1 may regulate vascular tone by stimulating production of nitric oxide synthase.[8] It is possible to increase cerebral perfusion in CFS patients with pharmacologic agents such as calcium channel blockers and acetazolamide (Diamox), but symptoms are not always relieved when this change occurs. Sometimes these medications fail to alter perfusion. This finding suggests that the regional hypoperfusion seen in CFS is an effect of an underlying pathophysiologic process, and also that the hypoperfusion is not the primary cause of the neurologic symptoms, although it may secondarily cause many of them. Anti-migraine drugs in general, such as ergotamine or beta blockers, have no particular beneficial effects in CFS. It will be interesting to try new medications to alter serotoninergic function such as sumatriptan and ondansetron. 5-HT neurons from the raphe nuclei diffusely innervate the cerebral vasculature, and fluoxetine (Prozac), which increases serotonin by specifically inhibiting its reuptake, seems to have some utility in CFS. Receptors for IL-1, as well as IL-1ra (*receptor antagonist*), an independently related cytokine, are present in dorsal raphe serotoninergic neurons. If IL-1ra is secreted in excess, stimulation of serotonin secretion could be impaired.[9] 5-HT receptor subtypes have both dilatory and constrictive effects on the cerebral vasculature, and the net effect on cerebral blood flow depends on the balance between contractile and relaxant receptors.[10] CO_2 tension and autonomic and neuropeptide function also help to regulate regional cerebral blood flow. An inhibition of the stimulation by IL-1 of nitric oxide synthase is the most parsimonious explanation of decreased regional cerebral blood flow in CFS.[11] A large number of endogenous and exogenous substances can alter cerebral blood flow[12], however. Neuropeptide Y is another candidate for causing CFS vasospasm, since its levels vary inversely with CRH.[13]

The fatigue of CFS, when not related to exertion, can be induced by stress, lack of sleep, or unknown causes. A broad range of changes occurs psychoneuroimmunologically when someone is exposed to stress. One common alteration is activation of the hypothalamic-pituitary-adrenal (HPA) axis. The hypercortisolemia seen in MDD is not seen in CFS, perhaps because there is decreased secretion of ACTH. Patients with CFS apparently have mildly abnormal CRH tests, and in my experience, ACTH stimulation tests sometimes do not produce the expected increase in plasma cortisol. Preliminary evidence suggests that urinary MHPG (a catecholamine metabolite) might not be increased in CFS, as it is in a subtype of MDD. There may be a central hypocortisolemia due to CRH deficiency, a possible unifying feature of the various neurasthenic states. CRH has a high concentration of receptors in the limbic system, where it also functions to regulate sympathetic tone, and has immunosuppressive effects independent of its stimulation of ACTH and cortisol.[14,15]

There must be some neurotransmitter mediation of the effects of stress or even mental exertion in CFS, but it is unclear which substance or its receptor might be deranged, although IL-1 beta is a candidate. I believe that repeated firing from the heterolimbic and paralimbic areas involved in stress or mental exertion could influence fatigue-inducing structures in the limbic zone. If 2,5A synthetase/RNase L production is also increased in the brain, ATP would be consumed in the process and neurons and glial cells thus would be less able to meet their energy needs. One or both mechanisms could be involved.

The alpha-EEG sleep abnormality described by Moldofsky in fibromyalgia patients is also seen in those with CFS.[16] Normal persons selectively deprived of slow-wave sleep developed fibromyalgia in one of his experiments. It is obvious clinically that sleep is often non-restorative in CFS and that if a patient does not get enough sleep one night his disease will often relapse.

The cause of the various CFS sleep disorders is unknown, although it is likely that limbic mechanisms are involved. IL-1 has been demonstrated to induce slow-wave (delta) sleep, and IL-1 and IL-2 levels increase during sleep. Although prefrontal structures may be dysfunctional, the region which generates alpha waves has not been certainly identified. How alpha waves disrupt slow-wave sleep is similarly unclear. A recent study by Moldofsky did not demonstrate normalization of sleep architecture when cyclobenzaprine (Flexeril) was administered to fibromyalgia patients, although some clinical improvement did occur.[17] The nature of the restorative function of sleep is far from obvious; with the preceding information one might wonder whether metabolism of accumulated cytokines would be involved. If cytokine production is excessive, or metabolism dysregulated, a patient could feel worse (as is often the case) when he wakes up than when he goes to bed. Eighty percent of growth hormone is secreted during stage 4 sleep. If this stage is disrupted, less somatomedin-C should be produced in the liver. Fibromyalgia patients have decreased levels of somatomedin-C as compared to controls,[18] another possible mechanism for fatigue and muscle pain due to impaired anabolism. Many times I have heard words to the effect of: "I woke up and felt like I had been hit by a train." As with many other components of CFS, the sleep disorder which accompanies CFS can be considered a cause, an effect, or some of both.

Fatigue is a common symptom associated with many medical disorders which needs to be considered when evaluating a patient. Common causes of fatigue include viral, infectious or inflammatory syndromes, endocrine disorders, and autoimmune diseases. Heart failure, chronic lung diseases, anemia, malabsorption, hepatic and renal failure all may be associated with fatigue due to inadequate delivery of nutrients and oxygen to various organ systems. Almost any chronic illness can cause fatigue, and neoplastic disorders should always be considered. Adverse drug reactions and ingestion of alcohol, toxins, or illicit substances may also produce fatigue. Sleep disorders are commonly overlooked as is chronic sinusitis, a fatigue-producing condition that should respond to proper therapy.

Depression, anxiety disorders, schizophrenia, and organic mental disorders can all be associated with fatigue, but the mechanism by which the fatigue is generated in these conditions is rarely addressed.

Neurologic disorders involving the skeletal muscle often produce weakness and fatigue, both symptoms of CFS. Myasthenia gravis, multiple sclerosis, post-polio syndrome, neuropathies, myopathies, and endocrine disorders should always be considered in this regard. Weakness and fatiguability on repetitive activity should be physiologically demonstrable in commonly used tests (such as dynamometry, ergometry, and electromyography). Such studies will not reliably show abnormalities in the CFS patient.

Cognitive Dysfunction

Cognitive dysfunction is now regarded as a hallmark of CFS and some well-known clinicians will not make the diagnosis of CFS unless intellectual impairment can be demonstrated. This deficit was not apparent to most early investigators and was still not prominently discussed at a consensus conference held at the National Institutes of Health in March, 1991. My impression of neuropsychological investigation that has been reported is that there are problems with quality control and precision of methodology, with some researchers reporting gross intellectual impairment, and others, none at all! Patients report significant difficulties with memory and concentration, and if testing instruments do not detect them, one is left with the possibility of a pseudodementia syndrome, in which patients complain of not being able to accomplish intellectual tasks of which they used to be capable. Research done by Curt Sandman, PhD, with my patients indicates that there is a specific type of CFS memory deficit.[19] CFS patients also usually overestimate their cognitive capabilities, unlike the depressed individual.

Patients with CFS have characteristic problems with the making of new memories, a process called "encoding." This is a distinctly hippocampal function, and CFS patients have the classic neuropsychologic profile of hippocampal lesioning. Their learning is very subject to interference, and of a particular kind: "proactive interference," when previously learned material interferes with the learning of new material, a process called "intrusion." In order to make a memory, a person must attend to a stimulus, screen out irrelevant stimuli, register and encode the stimulus (short-term memory), compare it to previous experiences and emotions, and then store it into long-term memory, from which it should be able to be retrieved. The process of turning short-term into long-term memory is termed consolidation. For the last decade, hippocampal encoding has been known to involve excitatory amino acids (EAAs) such as glutamate and aspartate. EAAs are also involved in seizure kindling and neuronal damage after anoxia or other insults.[20] It is unclear whether EAA agonists or antagonists would be beneficial in CFS; perhaps the problem is one of more subtle interrelationships between EAAs, cytokines, nerve growth factors, eicosanoids, neuropeptides, kinases, neurotransmitters, neurotoxic gene products, G proteins and nitric oxide (or other retrograde messengers).[21,22]

The process of making memories is very complex. Recent work indicates that secretion of endogenous benzodiazepines has an inhibitory effect on encoding and consolidation. If anxiety, which also produces interference, is present, endogenous benzodiazepines, acting allosterically at the $GABA_A$ receptor, could facilitate memory if secreted in sufficient amounts.[23] Exogenous benzodiazepines are now being administered to rats by microinjection into limbic structures to see their effect in various learning paradigms. Such research could also be done on CFS patients using short-acting systemic benzodiazepines such as alprazolam (Xanax). These patients often have general anxiety disorder/panic disorder, and even if they do not, subclinical deficits in endogenous benzodiazepines could affect memory without causing anxiety.

When EAA ligands that can pass the blood-brain barrier become available for clinical use, they may be valuable pharmacologic probes for the understanding and treatment of the CFS memory deficit. Common CFS patient complaints about short-term memory problems are the following:

1. "I walk into a room and forget why I went there."
2. "I need lists to remember everything –even lists of my lists."

3. "I can never remember what I read anymore, so I just watch TV; sometimes it's even hard to do that."

Dr. Sandman has done Auditory Evoked Response (AER) testing on patients with CFS and compared them with normals. The results of the patient group quite surprisingly segregate them markedly from normals. In assessing abnormalities in the AER (the electrical activity which occurs in the brain after an auditory stimulus is analyzed by a computer), a delay in neural transmission, indicating a lesion, is noted. All 12 CFS patients tested had abnormalities at the time the electrical activity should be going through the hippocampus, and none of the controls had such findings.[24]

Patients frequently complain of problems with attention and concentration. Attentional mechanisms are complex, involving a feedback circuit between the reticular activating system, the thalamic reticular nuclei, the parietal cortex, and the frontal lobes. As a stimulus loses its novelty, there is less input from the frontal lobes to maintain the activity of the attentional circuit, even though the unimodal sensory areas can still be shown to be firing. Norepinephrine and dopamine modulate this circuit, and stimulant drugs enhance attention by increasing levels of these neurotransmitters. Besides being easily distracted, another attentional disorder in CFS may be called "ideational apraxia," in which there is impairment of intent of the performance of complex motor tasks. Putting garbage in the refrigerator may be an example of such an impairment.

Stimulant drugs are not particularly effective in most patients with CFS, either for providing energy or enhancing concentration. Attentional deficits are somewhat difficult to demonstrate in a testing situation, except as fatigue supervenes. Thus the problem seems to be qualitatively different than in the individual with Attention Deficit Hyperactivity Disorder (ADHD), which has its onset in childhood and is associated with antisocial personality and substance abuse as an adult. The prefrontal hypoperfusion reported in SPECT scans of those with ADHD is, however, seen in CFS patients. Dorsolateral prefrontal lesions can induce a hypokinetic state.[25] Asymmetry or absence of the VER n-120 wave on the BEAM scan is frequent, however, and is thought by some to be a marker for attention deficit. Some children with ADD without hyperactivity may actually have CFS.[26]

The most common visual complaint in CFS patients is intermittent blurred vision, probably due to variations in the autonomic input to muscles which move the lens. Problems with accomodation are typical. Blurred vision often responds to nitroglycerin in very low doses. Nitroglycerin is metabolized into nitric oxide, a neurotransmitter which may be low in CFS (see Conclusion). Nystagmus has sometimes been detected by neuro-ophthalmologists at the University of Southern California School of Medicine, but is not frequently seen on a routine eye exam.[27] Photophobia is also a frequent complaint, and is probably due to ciliary muscle spasm. It can be treated to an extent with prostaglandin-inhibiting ophthalmic solution. Patients sometimes report that their concentration is impaired because the lines they are reading jump around and jumble. Some are unable to read for this reason. A less common, perhaps related complaint is that objects in the environment seem to move up and down, or back and forth. Oscillopsia may be seen with lesions of the vestibular nuclei, or in the parieto-occipital area. In the latter case, the illusion is present only in the contralateral homonymous visual field, not the finding in CFS. Night vision is also impaired, and is most troublesome when driving, when oncoming headlights appear overly bright. This phenomenon may be related to photophobia.

Other complaints are related to driving:

1. Inability to concentrate on a task. Both the hippocampus and the prefrontal cortex serve to filter and exclude irrelevant and interfering stimuli. With hippocampal damage, there is input overload which would disrupt the normal encoding process. The multiple stimuli to which one must attend or exclude during driving could be overwhelming and could also produce anxiety, if not appropriately processed.
2. Fear of driving alone. This is somewhat related to agoraphobia, since the patient feels better with someone else in the car.
3. Problems with spatial relations. The patient has difficulty judging distances between vehicles, or may get lost in his own neighborhood.

Spatial relation difficulties are frequently reported, yet are not reliably detected on neuropsychological tests administered to CFS patients. Topographic brain mapping by BEAM scanning in those with visual-spatial complaints often demonstrates a right parietal abnormality, perhaps in the inferior parietal lobule, which has limbic connections. I have found BEAM scanning generally useful in situations when neuropsychological testing could not demonstrate cognitive abnormalities based on cortical localization of function. Hippocampal lesions can produce "place" coding dysfunction in an animal who will be unsure about its spatial location.[28]

Dyscalculia is also frequently reported. Complaints by accountants of sometimes not being able to balance a checkbook are fairly common. Once again, parietal lobe lesions, left greater than right, are seen on the BEAM scan (the AERs and VERs are the most sensitive). The Gerstmann syndrome–dyscalculia, dysgraphia, finger identification disturbances and left-right naming difficulties–is rarely seen, nor are the various neglect syndromes. A small minority of CFS patients may have more widespread, extra-limbic neuronal dysfunction and may manifest such problems. They may occasionally be noted in Draw-A-Person tests when one side of the figure will be incompletely sketched. As with other cognitive deficits in CFS, the parietal lobe symptoms wax and wane, suggesting a transmitter-receptor mediated etiology, arterial spasm, or behavioral kindling. These sorts of patients have multifocal problems and sometimes have a testing profile like a patient with multi-infarct dementia.

Numerous other cognitive deficits are encountered in the CFS patient. A common problem is with planning and sequencing, the organization of the components of a complex task. This deficit may manifest itself by an inability to follow directions, perhaps not related to spatial relations, or by going to several locations while shopping. Following a recipe, or completing work-related assignments with multiple steps, can also be impaired. Planning and sequencing is thought to be a frontal lobe function.

Another disorder linked to frontal lobe dysfunction is difficulty with impulse control. Again, the indication of such an abnormality is best seen electrophysiologically by topographic brain mapping. CFS patients are not impulsive in the way that those with ADHD (Attention Deficit Hyperactivity Disorder) are, nor are they stimulus-seeking without regard for consequences in the manner of sociopaths. Rather, they can have periods of irritability, which often coincide with fatigue, in which normally placid individuals can become very angry and even throw things at loved ones.

Agnosias are fairly common. Visual agnosia means that an otherwise alert individual does not recognize a visual stimulus. This does not refer to being unable to name an object (anomia), another typical problem which does not have discrete cortical localization, but rather to not being able to recognize it. Occasionally a patient will have prosopagnosia, an inability to recognize human faces. Patients report not recognizing people whom they previously knew, which is distinct from not remembering their names, another common problem. Patients have even forgotten the names of their spouses or children. Prosopagnosias have been linked to bilateral lesions in visual association cortices. Recall that ictal foci in one limbic hemisphere can spread to the same site on the other side ("mirroring").

Associated with agnosias can be disorders of color perception. CFS patients perceive colors adequately and do not usually have problems with color naming, but color association may be impaired. It is quite striking when a patient relates that a traffic light can change from red to green and he forgets what that means.

Hearing loss is not usually seen in CFS, although patients may complain of not being able to hear well. On further questioning they will admit that the intensity of sound is adequate but that they are not able to discriminate words. Auditory discrimination may be a right parietal lobe function. If this area is abnormal on BEAM scanning I will sometimes ask a patient whether he has problems in auditory discrimination, and often the reply will be in the affirmative.

I should emphasize that lesions seen on the brain functional imaging may not cause behavioral or neurologic impairment, since the brain has a considerable reserve capacity. We assessed 12 patients with fibromyalgia and no subjective cognitive impairment. Neuropsychological testing showed some encoding problems, and BEAM scans demonstrated the same sort of temporal lobe lesions as are seen in CFS patients, but without as much spread into other cortical areas. Brain mapping in patients with severe IBS demonstrates a similar pattern. We have not done SPECT or PET scans in this population, but temporolimbic dysfunction seems probable.

CFS patients sometimes complain of slurred speech, particularly when fatigued. This dysarthria appears to be of the lower motor neuron type, as is seen in lesions of the lower pons or medulla. Since they do not seem to have cortical dysarthrias I can only speculate about how modulation of neural tone through descending tracts may cause this disorder. Slurred speech has been described, however, in temporolimbic epilepsy.

Psychiatric Disorders

The dementia of CFS is one of the primary patient complaints, but is not easily detected on mental status examination by neurologists, or by neuropsychological testing by some psychologists. It is not characteristic of the relatively "fixed" dementias seen in other organic mental disorders; some deficits are never seen, and CFS dementia symptoms wax and wane. Some very discrete and uncommon symptoms such as prosopagnosia or color association problems, which I had never heard of when I started seeing patients with CFS, have been described to me in an almost identical fashion by several patients. I now believe that if patients are told that their neuropsychological testing does not reveal any cognitive deficit then there is a problem with the instruments being used or with the sophistication of the psychologist's interpretation of the results. Just as an array of other "non-standard" tests will usually indicate dysfunction when a patient is told "you can't be sick–all your tests are normal," the right kind of neuropsychological tests, especially those for proactive interference, will usually be abnormal if they are done, but they are usually not part of standard test batteries.

Psychological problems in CFS patients either precede the onset of the illness or occur as a result of it. The latter difficulties may be present as a reaction to the limitations imposed by CFS. They may also be induced by the attitude of family and associates toward the patient. CFS can cause an organic mood disorder which is characterized by episodes of anxiety and/or depression, sometimes caused by general relapses, and other times unrelated to any apparent precipitants. Some patients appear to have a cyclothymic disorder. Borderline personality disorder is a diagnosis that may also be over-represented among those with CFS as compared to the healthy population.

There is some evidence that CFS patients with a pre-existing mood disorder have more severe symptoms and a poorer prognosis, although they do not differ in response to Ampligen. Minnesota Multiphasic Personality Inventory (MMPI) results compared with clinical symptoms by M. Yunus in a fibromyalgia patient population reveal that the more psychologically disturbed patients had more severe symptoms.[29] In this group one does not know whether the psychological disturbance was more of the endogenous variety that one would associate with a limbic encephalopathy, or was primarily reactive in nature. It would make sense that a pre-existing depressive disorder, since it can suggest a limbic dysfunction anyway, would be a marker for development of more severe CFS symptoms. Patients with severe depression may show loss of volume in the temporal lobes as determined by magnetic resonance imaging, suggesting a gliosis secondary to viral infection, oversecretion of cortisol, cell death from EAAs, or numerous other possible factors. Also seen in temporolimbic epilepsy and schizophrenia, this finding assuredly has prognostic significance. Since it is conceivable that mood disorders may be associated with viral limbic encephalitis, some patients could exhibit depressive symptomatology as the initial manifestation of a virally induced CFS which then emerged as a more complete syndrome as a result of subsequent immunodysfunctional influences.

Perhaps 20% of my patient population, which has a selection bias toward the more severe cases, report experiencing child abuse of some sort. This kind of stress on a developing, quite plastic nervous system could create a strong predisposition toward temporolimbic dysfunction and resultant somatic symptoms, much as are seen in patients with post-traumatic stress disorder (PTSD).[30] An increased incidence of childhood trauma is not found in patients with fibromyalgia, however.[31] It would be of interest to evaluate Vietnam veterans with PTSD for symptoms of CFS. Abused children are more likely to have several sorts of problems as adults. Borderline personality disorder is one of them, but others, e.g., drug dependence and multiple personality disorder, are not more common in the CFS population than in normals. There is one study that reports an increased incidence of drug dependence in patients with chronic fatigue (not chronic fatigue *syndrome*).[32]

Patients with CFS may have a lowered self-esteem and a sensitivity to rejection. They usually are quite upset over their inability to perform tasks as they could premorbidly, and may have a decreased financial and social support system. Husbands have beaten their wives because they thought they were lazy, and divorces have occurred because the spouse did not understand the illness and/or could not handle the pressures of living with a person who had a chronic, disabling illness which could not be authentically demonstrated to much of the medical profession. The general public, relatives, friends, and neighbors may be afraid of "catching it." Patients may withdraw from social interactions not just because of fatigue, but because friends do not understand CFS, and the patient gets tired of making up excuses for unavailability.

The irritability that CFS patients have is usually intermittent. Some patients relate it to frustration with the illness, and others cannot understand it. "Rage attacks" with violent lashing out are not infrequent. Certain medications for treatment of rage attacks (lithium, propanolol) are not effective, but others (buspirone, fluoxetine) may be. As with other CFS symptoms, if the entire syndrome improves, so does the irritability.

The incidence of anxiety and panic disorder is increased in CFS patients, and agoraphobia while driving is encountered frequently. Patients are more prone to have panic attacks when they are relapsing. A condition of panic attacks without fear should be considered when assessing patient symptomatology.[33,34] The jury is still out as to whether panic attacks are a form of temporolimbic epilepsy. They can be successfully treated with clonazepam (Klonopin) and valproic acid (Depakote) but not very well with carbamazepine (Tegretol). Many authorities implicate the locus ceruleus, the noradrenergic projection center for the brain, with extensive projections to the limbic system, as the generator of panic attacks.[35] Some would even place the locus ceruleus in the limbic system. Others have found limbic PET scan abnormalities in panic disorder patients,[36] although these findings have recently been attributed to spasm in the temporalis muscle secondary to bruxism.[37]

Five percent of my patients have a bipolar I or II disorder. Many of these are somewhat treatment-resistant, and some have had their bipolar diagnosis well treated but still have all the other symptoms of CFS. These patients' moods are often quite sensitive to IVIG (intravenous immunoglobulin). A few of them have had mania precipitated by infusions and were not able to tolerate the medication. Perhaps IVIG has an anti-idiotypic action in these patients as well as, or instead of, the cytokine modulatory effect that I assume is operative in most individuals. IVIG may also block antibodies to various transmitters, thereby increasing the functional activity of the transmitters. Bipolar disorders, perhaps more than any other psychiatric diagnostic category, are believed to have a limbic etiology. Some of these patients respond well to nitroglycerin, but higher doses are often required than for the usual CFS patient.

A neuroanatomic or neurophysiologic localization for borderline personality disorder is currently obscure. I have had a much larger number of such patients in my practice since I began specializing in CFS, and the psychiatric disorder has antedated the rest of the symptoms in all concerned. These patients are the most difficult to manage. Working in a medical model as I do becomes especially challenging when no medical therapy is effective. It is difficult to treat borderline CFS patients without a concomitant psychotherapist, since it is hard to "change gears" to adopt the sort of supportive, limit-setting psychotherapeutic posture that is advocated for management. Another difficulty is the fact that a busy CFS practice may have 15 or 20 borderlines at any one time. This patient mix is extremely demanding in both time and stress and would be daunting to even the most skillful physician. A sizable number of patients were diagnosed as being borderline prior to seeing me. I have found them to be dissatisfied and frustrated people with reactive depressions who do not fit well into the common diagnostic scheme. If I am able to improve their CFS symptoms, the emotional lability and other features that characterize these supposed borderlines are ameliorated to varying degrees.

Schizophrenic patients are uncommon in a CFS practice. When I do see one, the presenting complaint is usually fatigue along with schizophrenic symptoms. It is very unusual to see the complete chronic fatigue syndrome in a schizophrenic patient. Since both disorders involve abnormalities in the medial temporal lobe, I must assume that different neurochemical tracts are involved,[38] especially since neuroleptic or dopaminergic agents are rarely of value in CFS. When I consult with a fatigued schizophrenic, I always wonder whether he might have temporolimbic epilepsy (TLE) without the classic symptoms since schizophreniform psychosis has frequently been described in this disorder. Many CFS patients have TLE, and I always give a trial of anticonvulsant medication to see whether I can improve the symptoms of the fatigued schizophrenic patient. Some fatigued schizophrenics appear encephalopathic on brain functional imaging and have the same encoding problems as do patients with CFS.

Other psychiatric disorders are rarely encountered. In particular, obsessive-compulsive disorder and Tourette's syndrome are hardly ever seen, suggesting that the limbic striatum may be fairly intact. We do, however, see lesions in the limbic striatum on PET scan, and the anterior caudate nucleus is commonly hypometabolic. It may be beyond the limits of current PET resolution to image structures in the limbic striatum such as the nucleus accumbens.

The mesotelencephalic dopaminergic systems which lack autoreceptors, the mesoprefrontal and mesocingulate, could possibly be involved in CFS. These systems do not respond well to agonists or antagonists, but since they have a high metabolic rate, may be differentially affected by precursors such as tyrosine.[39] Monoamine oxidase inhibitors (MAOIs) may preferentially target such receptors which could explain their efficacy in treatment-resistant depression and possibly CFS, although the latter result might be related to an effect on the mitochondrial membrane. Beta-endorphin and other endogenous opioids may stimulate mu-2 receptors in these areas to enhance dopamine release.[40]

I used to think that alcoholics could not get CFS, since it was difficult to make the diagnosis in a patient who did not have alcohol intolerance of some sort. This rule is not hard and fast, however, since I have a few recovering alcoholics in my practice. Drug seeking behavior is not frequently seen, either. Most patients in whom I would diagnose drug dependence also have borderline personality disorder. Sociopathy is quite rare, as is attention deficit disorder with hyperactivity. I hypothesize that these conditions have a completely different anatomic substrate than the limbic encephalopathy of CFS.

Developmental learning disorders are encountered more frequently in the CFS population, particularly reading disorders. Most of these patients do not have a history of a CFS-like problem as children, so one must assume either a defect in neuronal maturation or migration, or a mild viral encephalopathy which could have caused a learning disorder and could have possibly "set the stage" for CFS in the future.

Eating disorders may be slightly over-represented in the CFS population, although anorexia nervosa and bulimia nervosa are fairly widespread disorders in the general population. It is probably fortunate that they do not occur more frequently in CFS, because many patients have a marked, rapid weight gain. An increase of fifty pounds in six months is not uncommon. One patient I saw recently claimed to have gained fifty-six pounds in six weeks! What would this do to an eating disorder patient with a distorted body image?

Hysterical disorders are not common and only two of my patients have had multiple personality disorder. Dissociative disorders or fugue states which also occur more frequently in victims of child abuse could be subsumed under temporal lobe phenomena. Hypochondriacs present much less frequently than would be expected, although they may come to the office of the CFS practitioner in their long search for help. Inquiring of these patients about temporolimbic symptoms should be done but it is rarely productive. It is not difficult for me to distinguish the patient with somatization disorder from one with CFS. Patients with somatization disorder should not have recurrent flu-like illnesses with sore throat, specific encoding problems, fibromyalgia tender points, laboratory results suggesting immune activation, or characteristic findings on brain functional imaging. The symptoms of somatization disorder must begin prior to age 30 in order to be diagnosed by DSM-III-R criteria. The average age of onset of CFS is the mid-30s. I thus find patients with somatization disorder to be rare, although the diagnosis is made frequently.

Sleep Disorders

It is difficult to make the diagnosis of CFS if a patient does not have certain sleep disorders. The ones that present most frequently are, in order of incidence:

1. Disorder of Initiating and Maintaining Sleep (DIMS)
2. Hypersomnia
3. Sleep-Phase Disorder
4. Bruxism (grinding the teeth)
5. Restless Legs Syndrome (RLS) and Periodic Limb Movements During Sleep (PLMS), also called Nocturnal Myoclonus
6. Nightmares or extremely vivid dreams
7. Night sweats or other disorders of thermoregulation
8. Frequent awakenings due to nocturia
9. Nocturnal panic attacks
10. Sleep apnea

Most CFS sleep is non-restorative.

DIMS is far and away the most common CFS sleep disorder. An inability to fall asleep even though exhausted ("wired and tired") with frequent wakenings is the usual story. This type of DIMS may be called persistent psychophysiological insomnia and is usually attributed to poor sleep hygiene, worrying too much, or alternatively, to generalized anxiety disorder. The DIMS of CFS does not seem to fit well into any of these categories. The patients do not usually worry about being able to fall asleep and sleeping is usually not better when they sleep in a different environment. Patients often fall asleep when not trying to sleep. The DIMS does not usually begin during a period of stress, unless a prolongation of CFS could be termed an inciting stress. Patients whose illness begins with an acute flu-like episode usually manifest hypersomnia, which then becomes DIMS after a while. Some patients alternate between DIMS and hypersomnia. It appears to me that CFS DIMS is caused by the disease, and that there is a physiologic abnormality in the control of sleep onset and maintenance. The mechanisms which generate sleep and wakefulness are highly complex from a neurophysiologic and neurochemical point of view. The neurologic factors involved in DIMS are quite unknown, and have not been well studied.

Idiopathic central nervous system hypersomnia is characterized by long, undisturbed nocturnal sleep, daytime drowsiness which impairs performance, sleep drunkenness when awakening, and automatic behavior. Sleep attacks as seen in narcolepsy are not too common and when they occur, are not present in REM sleep.

CFS patients have all the symptoms of this disorder except for sleep drunkenness, which is rare. Automatic behavior, such as putting garbage in the refrigerator or finding oneself miles away from a planned destination, is fairly common and can be hard to distinguish from ideomotor apraxia, fugue states, or temporolimbic epilepsy. None of my hypersomnic CFS patients has had polysomnography, but sleep architecture in idiopathic hypersomnia is not different from normals, just longer. Christian Guilleminault has divided idiopathic central nervous system hypersomnia into three subgroups:[41]

1. Those with a positive family history and expression of the HLACw2 antigen (narcoleptics are more likely to express HLADR2). Autonomic abnormalities such as Raynaud's disorder are common in this population. CFS patients may have an increase in HLADR4, but not Cw2. Other researchers have found no abnormalities in CFS HLA typing.
2. As a post-viral syndrome, either after mononucleosis or viral pneumonia. Patients in this group will also complain of being fatigued. (Sound familiar?)
3. Idiopathic. Guilleminault notes that this disorder is poorly understood and poorly controlled by medical therapy.

Sleep phase disorders are grouped under the heading of Disorders of the Sleep-Wake Schedule (DSWS). CFS patients are very sensitive to chronobiologic, or circadian, disruption. Jet lag and shift work cause greater difficulty than in the normal population. CFS patients often show phase advance, wanting to fall asleep earlier, or phase delay, wanting to fall asleep later. Circadian rhythms are determined to a great extent by the suprachiasmatic nucleus (SCN) in the hypothalamus.[42] I am not aware of any direct extrahypothalamic innervation of the SCN, although it is well known to be regulated by the retinal-hypothalamic and geniculo-hypothalamic tract. Other neural inputs come from within the hypothalamus. Regulation of melatonin secretion from the pineal gland is determined by the SCN. Melatonin determines synchronization of endocrine organs and has immunomodulatory properties mediated, at least in part, by stimulation of endogenous opioids released by antigen-activated T-helper lymphocytes. Exogenous melatonin can alleviate jet lag and synchronize other biological rhythms. Affective and psychosomatic illnesses have been associated with altered patterns of melatonin secretion. Variations in melatonin secretory rhythms have not been reported in CFS. The assay is experimental and the substance is secreted in a pulsatile manner during darkness in normal subjects although this pattern of secretion may be deranged in various disease states. Melatonin is highly concentrated in the SCN, suggesting a feedback mechanism. Because of the description of circadian physiology in CFS and the waxing and waning of symptomatology in the disease without external cues, melatonin research would be important. There is a reciprocal relationship between vitamin D and melatonin.[43] My measurements of 1,25 dihydroxy vitamin D in CFS have been normal, even in those with marked sunlight intolerance. If there were melatonin abnormalities, I might expect to see them reflected in vitamin D levels.

Temperature regulation, a preoptic and anterior hypothalamic function, is related to sleep physiology. Metabolic rate in rats, as measured by heat production, is higher during the awake state than in REM sleep, and higher in NREM than in REM sleep. In humans, metabolic rate in REM is greater than NREM. This difference is thought to be related to the much greater cortical surface in humans, and that cerebral blood flow is greater during REM than NREM. Sweating during sleep, a common CFS complaint, is more common during Slow-Wave Sleep stages 3 and 4 except during bursts of REM associated with dreaming. Since CFS patients have very vivid dreams, it is not possible to say in which sleep stage the sweating occurs. Slow-wave sleep is characteristically disrupted in CFS ("alpha-EEG" sleep) and this alteration could cause more sympathetic arousal which could produce sweating.

Sleep and basal temperature rhythms have a complex interaction. If sleep can become uncoupled from temperature regulation, as it can during prolonged isolation from temporal cues, DIMS may occur. Temperature must be falling in order for a person to go to sleep. Although this parameter has not been investigated (to my knowledge) in CFS, patients feel hot and/or cold so often that this specific disorder of thermoregulation might be possible.

Both the delayed and advanced sleep phase syndrome are usually treated with chronotherapy or bright light therapy. In chronotherapy, the patient takes time off from work and goes to sleep three hours later each night. He then stops this process when he arrives at the hour that he would desire sleep onset. I must say that this procedure has never worked in my CFS patients and often makes them relapse, since getting as good a night's sleep as possible is essential. In sleep phase disorders the sleep architecture is usually normal, and thus CFS patients could not strictly be said to have such problems. I vividly recall one woman, however, who was so entrained to her sleep phase that when her workplace altered her hours so that she would begin work one or two hours earlier, she developed both CFS and an intractable sleep disorder. When she would take a week or two off and sleep from 11 p.m. to 7 a.m. she recovered, but after returning to work, lying in bed awake from 9 to 11 p.m., falling asleep at 11 p.m., but waking up at 5 a.m. always caused her to relapse. She did not recover and eventually had to quit her job. A worker's compensation claim is pending.

CFS patients also have irregular sleep-wake patterns. They are unable to sleep for one long period, but must sleep in several periods. Their total sleep time is normal, differing from DIMS in that respect (DIMS causes a reduced 24-hour sleep time). Patients with DIMS usually have difficulty napping, while CFS patients usually must do so. Patients with somatoform disorders usually have DIMS as well, with difficulty napping.

Restless legs syndrome (RLS) and periodic limb movements during sleep (PLMS) are commonly seen in CFS, as they are in fibromyalgia, diabetes mellitus, uremia, anemia, rheumatoid arthritis, and leukemia. The etiology of these conditions is unknown, although they may occur in families. RLS consists of dysesthesias in both legs accompanied by irresistible urges to move them. Symptoms occur mainly at rest. The main differential diagnosis is akathisia, although dysesthesias are not commonly reported in this condition.

PLMS used to be called nocturnal myoclonus. The great toe extends and the foot dorsiflexes. Sometimes there is flexion of the knee and thigh as well. PLMS can occur with periodicity during sleep and occurs primarily during stage 1 and 2 sleep. There may be reduced stage 3 and 4 sleep. RLS and PLMS may be related to disinhibition of reticular excitability. They are commonly seen in association with other processes that can disrupt the sleep-wake schedule. PLMS is often reported by a spouse and is a fairly common disturbance. Some patients complain that "when I wake up in the morning I feel like I have run a marathon." It should always be suspected in the patient who has insomnia.

Bruxism is another sleep disorder of unknown cause common in CFS, and may also have a genetic proclivity. It is seen very frequently in those with fibromyalgia. Bruxism is encountered frequently in the general population; ten percent would be a conservative estimate. It can occur in REM and NREM sleep but is not destructive during REM sleep. Bruxism occurs in various types of encephalopathy, stress, in patients taking L-dopa or amphetamines, and in some patients with malocclusion. Sleep apnea and PLMS are also associated. Bruxism can cause development of trigger points in the masseter, medial and lateral pterygoids, and temporalis muscles, producing the temporomandibular pain and dysfunction syndrome (TMPDS) common in CFS. Dopaminergic tracts are thought to be involved, and bruxism is thought to be caused by disinhibition which is poorly understood. The anatomic localization of the dysfunction is not known, but may be in the amygdala (see Chapter 6).

Acroparesthesias are also frequently described by those with CFS and are usually bilateral, making pressure neuropathies unlikely. They are fairly constant, unlike the acroparesthesias of hyperventilation syndrome. Carpal tunnel syndrome is increased in frequency in CFS, but in my experience is not the most common cause of acroparesthesia since there is often paresthesia or hypesthesia of the feet as well. Tarsal tunnel syndrome is not a common disorder. I believe the acroparesthesias in CFS have a thalamic etiology. Some patients with very severe acroparesthesias have multiple sclerosis.

There are numerous other causes for sleep fragmentation which may be somewhat more common in the CFS patient. Panic attacks are almost certainly more frequent in this population, as is gastroesophageal reflux disease and obstructive sleep apnea. Common complaints, probably more directly related to the limbic system, are vivid dreams and violent, graphic nightmares.

Dreaming occurs during REM sleep. In depression, there is increased REM density (and probably more dreaming). CFS has not produced any particular alteration in REM sleep. Dreaming occurs when a group of neurons in the pons, near the reticular formation and the junction with the midbrain, begin to fire (pontogeniculate-occipital, or PGO "spikes"). They project into the visual areas and thus dreams occur. Visual association areas are numerous, and would include heteromodal and paralimbic areas. If the paralimbic areas are dysfunctional, dream content would be altered. If the modulation by the reticular formation of the PGO spikes were disrupted, dream content might be more vivid. The hippocampus is also tonically active during REM sleep, generating synchronized theta waves.[44] Patients who sleep less deeply are more apt to remember their dreams. Those with DIMS should therefore be more likely to be aware of them. A hippocampal dysfunction in CFS could also alter dream content by altered modulation of paralimbic and heteromodal afferents. REM sleep deprivation causes hyperactivity of several limbic structures.

The fact that sleep is non-restorative could be due to the alpha-EEG sleep abnormality. In order to diagnose alpha-EEG sleep, one must have an epoch of 5 to 20 percent of delta waves interspersed with high amplitude alpha-like rhythms. Patients with alpha-EEG sleep have a number of medical and psychiatric disorders. Alpha-EEG sleep can occupy a large percentage (up to 45 percent) of sleep time. It has been suggested that the non-restorative nature of alpha-EEG sleep may be due to suppression of nocturnal growth hormone secretion, which occurs during NREM sleep.

The cause of alpha-EEG sleep abnormality in CFS and fibromyalgia (FM) is unknown. Numerous neurotransmitters, neuropeptides, and cytokines are involved in sleep onset and maintenance, and the location of a specific population of alpha-generating neurons which could cause this disorder is uncertain although an alpha rhythm has recently been described in the temporal neocortex. The transmitters or neurons invoked are also unknown, although the alpha waves in CFS may be due to inappropriate alerting during slow-wave sleep or inadequate suppression of activity in the temporal neocortex. Limbic dysfunction could obviously be implicated. Alpha rhythm has been related to decreased melatonin secretion by the pineal gland,[45] an abnormality which is compatible with CFS pathophysiology. Patients with panic disorder are said by Katon[46] to be more aware of physiologic alterations in their internal milieu than normals, and perhaps the same could be said about CFS patients, although this increased awareness could be related to dysfunction of the insula and amygdala. It has been suggested by anatomical mapping with horseradish peroxidase that "connections between the insular cortical fields may be important for the integration of visceral sensation with ongoing behavior and autonomic response."[47] Such a mechanism may be the neurobiologic basis for "somatosensory amplification" to be discussed in a subsequent chapter. Other paralimbic areas may have a similar role. Limbic regulation of SWS is rather complex, and parallels the regulation of autonomic balance. The caudate nucleus and orbitofrontal cortex are said to promote cortical EEG synchrony and behavioral sleep, and to balance the sleep-suppressing activity of the caudal diencephalon and rostral brain stem. The activity of the midbrain reticular formation is modulated by the septum, amygdala, and orbitofrontal cortex, and these regions also direct projections to the nucleus of the solitary tract and the pontine parabrachial nuclei.

Headache is a common CFS symptom. Although there are several kinds of headaches, the most common is the tension-type headache. Next might be a pressure-type headache that is sometimes relieved by acetazolamide (Diamox). One might expect migraine headaches to be frequent in this population, as they are in other disorders of autonomic regulation, and that is the case. Sinus or allergy headaches, which many authorities believe are overdiagnosed, seem to be fairly prevalent in CFS. On the other hand, I have never seen a CFS patient with cluster headache or temporal (cranial) arteritis, although I have seen an occasional individual with an apparent mild lupus cerebritis who was seronegative but had a gadolinium-enhanced MRI of the brain which appeared to show a vasculitis. Sometimes the salivary glands will also light up, even though Sjogren antibodies will be absent.

If one looks for the characteristic tender points of fibromyalgia, the trigger points of tension headache, or the masseter and temporalis tenderness of TMPDS, they will almost always be present. Patients with maxillary sinus pain may have trigger points in the lateral pterygoid to explain their pain when sinus imaging is normal. Many do have sinusitis, often unexpectedly, and the treatment of the sinusitis has been reported to relieve many CFS symptoms (usually not, however, in my practice). Sometimes a patient will have pseudotumor cerebri, or benign intracranial hypertension. There may be forme frustes of this syndrome, since the "pressure" headaches do respond to Diamox frequently. The cause of pseudotumor cerebri is unknown, although IL-1 receptors are found in the choroid plexus.[48] Could pseudotumor be caused by an excessive manufacture of cerebrospinal fluid? In general, however, it would appear that the headaches of CFS are caused by a type of descending pain modulation disorder that has been suggested for fibromyalgia.

As has been mentioned previously, disturbances in visual acuity are common in CFS. They include problems with accommodation causing intermittent blurred vision and photophobia, probably due to ciliary muscle spasm since it is treatable with ocular prostaglandin inhibitors. The common complaint of oscillopsia could be due to brain stem dysfunction, since subtle nystagmus is sometimes seen, or may be related to difficulty with fixation, which could produce the phenomenon of lines of print jumping around while reading. Most of these visual disturbances are caused by autonomic dysfunction, perhaps again secondary to limbic-hypothalamic dysregulation. Neuro-ophthalmologic exam is usually normal, although nystagmus has been reported in 27% of patients in one series.[49]

Tinnitus and vertigo are common CFS complaints. The tinnitus is almost always bilateral and is not accompanied by hearing loss. The vertigo gets worse as symptoms increase. Sophisticated neuro-otologic testing has not revealed any consistent pattern in CFS patients with vertigo. The most severe vertigo is caused by end-organ damage. A minority of CFS vertigo patients have evidence of endolymphatic hydrops and perilymphatic fistula, perhaps secondary to benign intracranial hypertension. The rest seem to have a more central etiology for their symptoms. CFS vertigo is intermittent. For this reason a brain stem or more rostral source for the complaint is possible, since accommodation to unilateral lesions occurs as a matter of course. Even a complete section of one vestibular nerve will cause severe vertigo for only 6 months or so. There are so many inputs to central pathways mediating balance that it is difficult to lesion them all. Perhaps the intermittent nature of CFS vertigo does not allow tolerance to develop. If there is a temporolimbic focus it may elicit a "mirror" lesion in the other hemisphere which could contribute to chronicity. Vestibulospinal testing by platform posturography will sometimes show abnormalities of the postural control system. Pontine nuclei, including the locus ceruleus, project to the cerebellum. Centers in the cerebellum project to vestibular areas and could produce vestibular symptoms. Nystagmus can sometimes be detected in these patients but caloric testing is usually normal. Vertigo is sometimes associated with temporolimbic epilepsy but is not believed to present from a temporal lobe focus independently of a seizure disorder. Given the frequency of vertigo in the CFS patients, I must question this dogma. Tonal tinnitus may also have extra-cochlear etiologies. The pathophysiology of some of them, such as cervical spine disease, is obscure. Tinnitus has rarely been reported as a result of temporal lobe lesions, and a pathway from the temporal lobe to the cochlea has been suggested.

Temporolimbic epilepsy was discussed previously. Although it is not rampant among CFS patients, the incidence of this seizure disorder in CFS is probably greater than in the normal population. Temporolimbic epilepsy is probably underdiagnosed. The electrical activity of the medial temporal lobes and other limbic regions, including the insula, cingulate gyrus, and orbitofrontal cortex, is inaccessible to standard EEG leads and sometimes to specially placed electrodes such as nasopharyngeal and sphenoid leads. It would be incorrect to describe most phenomena in CFS as being examples of temporolimbic epilepsy, since they do not have symptoms in the regular, stereotyped nature associated with seizure disorder.

Many of the behavioral aspects of temporolimbic ictal phenomena should be familiar to those who deal with CFS. These have been discussed by M-Marsel Mesulam and others in *Principles of Behavioral Neurology*. Sensory alterations include tingling, numbness, or crawling dysesthesias which are in no known anatomic pattern.

Stuttering or slurred speech, even complete speech arrest, can occur. Autonomic manifestations include flushing, which may be regional, dyspnea, weight on the chest, air hunger, chest pain, palpitations, and sinus tachycardia. Nausea, or epigastric distress, is said to be the most common autonomic symptom.

An interictal behavioral disorder consisting of obsessive-compulsive behavior, hypergraphia, hyperreligiosity, emotional clinging, hyposexuality, and other traits has been associated with temporolimbic epilepsy and has been suggested for inclusion in the *Diagnostic and Statistical Manual of Mental Disorders,* fourth edition (DSM-IV). Many individuals do not manifest these behaviors at all, and they are uncommon in CFS. Some patients with dissociative disorders or atypical affective illness may show some response to anticonvulsants, even if seizure disorder cannot be demonstrated. The diagnosis of temporolimbic dysfunction, or "dysrhythmia," is quite controversial at this time, since it expands the concept of the symptoms of deranged limbic electrophysiology beyond the boundaries of what is accepted by many neurologists. Amplification of the notion of "behavioral kindling," as described by Robert Post, may help to bridge this gap in understanding, especially since manic-depressive and schizoaffective illness respond to certain anticonvulsants, as does panic disorder. Limbic, especially hippocampal, neurons are the most sensitive to kindling. Limbic and thalamic kindling may be inhibited by serotoninergic agents.[50] In the epilepsy model of amygdala-kindled seizures, repeated intermittent subconvulsant electrical stimuli in an animal result in the appearance of spontaneous seizures. Previously subthreshold experiential stimuli can eventually evoke robust behavioral phenomena, a process called "behavioral kindling."[51]

Some CFS patients feel very weak when they are relapsing. If they are extremely ill they feel weak all the time and have difficulty walking. Neurologic exam and electrophysiologic testing usually do not reveal any cause for the weakness. I believe the cause of the weakness is central, like the fatigue (in most cases). When patients have sleep drunkenness, they are sometimes weak. Whatever causes the sleep-drunkenness type of weakness may be similar to the cause of CFS weakness. An example of a similar type of periodic weakness is that seen in narcolepsy, but definite muscular atony can be demonstrated in this disorder as a result of the descending inhibition of motor pathways seen in REM sleep.

Many patients have fasciculations of muscle, a few to an alarming degree. Few have atrophy, persistent weakness, or reflex changes, as may be seen in other disorders which can cause fasciculation, particularly motor neuron diseases such as amyotrophic lateral sclerosis. Benign fasciculations may be due to hyperirritability of motor neuronal membranes, perhaps related to a disorder of descending modulation.

Recurrent flu-like illnesses with sore throat are one of the distinguishing characteristics of CFS. Recurrent sore throats are unusual manifestations of systemic illness but have been reported in autoimmune disorders such as rheumatic fever. The presence of this symptom complex in the majority of patients is a major argument for CFS being a cytokine-mediated illness. However, some patients who show laboratory evidence of chronic immune activation do not develop these flu-like illnesses, suggesting that in these cases there may be an unusual resistance to viral infection as a result of heightened immune surveillance.

There is ample evidence that limbic dysfunction can affect immune regulation. Much of it has been discussed previously. Since the brain and the immune system are an integrated unit, it is difficult to assign primacy to one area in the recurrent flu of CFS. The striking association of flu symptoms with stress and physical and mental exertion in CFS strongly argues for a limbic regulation of this condition, perhaps by central and/or peripheral secretion of IL-1.

It has become almost axiomatic that allergies, especially nasal allergy, are associated with CFS. Many patients who later develop CFS have nasal allergy, and those who have CFS note that their allergic symptoms get worse or that they develop them for the first time. Although it is known that mucosal mast cells are individually innervated, as are certain eosinophils, the limbic control of mast cell function has not been addressed. The parasympathetic innervation of the nose arises from the superior salivatory nucleus of the brain stem, with synaptic interruption in the sphenopalatine ganglion, and with distribution of post-ganglionic fibers to the nose, nasopharynx, and larynx. Parasympathetic stimulation in CFS could thus be responsible for an increase in nasal secretions, sore throat, and hoarseness, with release of the appropriate transmitter substances. Dysfunction of the glossopharyngeal nerve may account for most throat pain. Limbic innervation, particularly amygdalar innervation of the superior salivatory nucleus, could thus affect these structures. Allergic nasal secretions have been found to contain somatostatin, calcitonin gene-related peptide (CGRP), substance P, and histamine.[52] Since there is ample anecdotal evidence that successful treatment of allergic rhinitis (and sinusitis) can produce improvement in CFS, one may postulate a retrograde axonal mechanism, possibly involving transport of mediators, to explain this relationship. Inhaled substances that contact the nasal epithelium may cross into the brain.[53] If the nose and throat are irritated, receptors in the nose and sinuses communicate with afferent fibers of the trigeminal nerve. Collaterals from trigeminal nerve fibers enter the dorsal vagal nucleus and may travel cephalad to enter the diencephalon, or caudally, to cause reflex bronchoconstriction. Nasal epithelial damage occurs from inappropriate release of mediators from mast cells and eosinophils. There may be limbic mediation of this release.

Weight loss in some patients and rapid weight gain in others does not seem to be mediated by changes in appetite. A decrease in activity due to fatigue may contribute to weight gain, but would not cause a 50-pound weight gain in 8 weeks or so as has been reported by some patients. From what I know today about weight regulation, brown fat thermogenesis must be involved.[54] Brown Adipose Tissue (BAT) which dissipates caloric intake by heat, has beta adrenergic innervation. Other transmitter substances are involved as well, including CGRP, substance P, bombesin, and other neuropeptides. Limbic hypothalamic regulation of BAT sympathetic neurons could explain these rapid weight fluctuations. Rats infected with Borna virus, which has tropism for limbic and hypothalamic structures, become quite obese.[55] The central control of BAT thermogenesis in man is not well understood. It has been studied primarily in rats and Syrian hamsters. The CNS, by an unknown mechanism, can regulate control of sympathetic neural input to individual structures, such as BAT, without altering general sympathetic tone. Neurotransmitters have been implicated in the central control of BAT, notably corticotropin releasing hormone (CRH). CRH levels in CFS are probably decreased and weight loss is not a common chronic complaint.

Drug companies are hard at work to develop agents that will selectively activate BAT. One route might be by stimulating a novel adrenergic receptor found only in BAT, the beta-3 receptor. As of now, the safest available agent to use in CFS which activates BAT is fenfluramine (Pondimin), a serotonin agonist. I have investigated this drug in CFS obesity. Fenfluramine also increases CRH secretion. It should be used with some caution, however, since D-fenfluramine has been reported to cause neuronal degeneration.[56]

The cause of irritable bowel syndrome (IBS) is complex, but almost certainly invokes the limbic system. Some studies suggest that panic disorder and numerous other CFS symptoms common to CFS occur in association with IBS. Our work in functional brain imaging in IBS patients reveals abnormalities similar to those seen in CFS patients, although we have a much smaller sample of IBS patients. Descending influences on vagal nuclei from the limbic system could well be involved. There has also been degeneration of the myenteric plexus reported in an IBS patient who had a 95% colectomy for obstipation.[57] IBS has been relieved by administration of leuprolide acetate (Lupron), a gonadotropin-releasing hormone (GnRH) agonist used in the treatment of prostatic cancer and endometriosis.[58] Cells which stain for GnRH have been found in sympathetic ganglia and the bladder as well as in the limbic system. Neuronal projections from the lateral hypothalamus, insular cortex, solitary tract, and amygdaloid nuclei project directly to sympathetic preganglionic areas and could be affected by GnRH agonists. Lupron also has immunosuppressive actions, primarily on B lymphocytes, and is being used in clinical trials for this purpose. The possibility that a virus which could have a neurotoxic effect on limbic and myenteric structures by expression of a gene product, thus causing an encephalopathy/enteric neuropathy which would be non-inflammatory, could be considered as a possible etiologic factor. Retroviruses may act in this manner, and a human foamy virus has been reported to cause hippocampal as well as intestinal smooth muscle degeneration in transgenic mice.[59]

IBS patients have a high incidence of fibromyalgia, Raynaud's syndrome, and fatigue. Many of them are similar to CFS patients although some have primarily gastrointestinal symptoms or symptoms of idiopathic intestinal hollow visceral neuropathy. Since the myenteric plexus as well as the limbic system may be dysfunctional in these patients, food intolerance (not allergies) and development of bizarre postprandial symptoms could be explained by deranged release of transmitter substances from the enteric nervous system, by afferent neural transmission via the vagus and splanchnic nerves to the nucleus of the solitary tract, amygdala, and to the hypothalamic lateral and paraventricular nuclei. Neurotransmitter precursors such as tryptophan, tyrosine, and phenylalanine are also transported to the brain, and there are postprandial CSF increases in alpha fibroblast growth factor and insulin.[60] CSF CRH has been reported to increase post-prandially, perhaps related to why some CFS patients feel better after eating.[61] Dietary recommendations for patients with IBS include a low tyramine diet and avoidance of red meat, since enteric and CNS receptors may be dysregulated, and migraine headaches may be more common in this population as well. IBS is often noted to begin after a viral illness.

Patients with food intolerance can be diagnosed and treated with an elimination diet. This technique can be used whether or not the intolerance is IgE-mediated. The symptoms and diseases that may signify reactions to foods[62] overlap with chronic fatigue syndrome. The mechanism of these varied reactions to food is not well understood, yet could involve limbic mechanisms.

Fibromyalgia

The etiology of fibromyalgia (FM) is still unknown. A defect in muscle microcirculation has been found fairly consistently, perhaps causing hypoxia. Non-restorative sleep due to the alpha-EEG sleep abnormality is common. There is a possibility that CNS metabolism of serotonin, catecholamines, and substance P is dysregulated. Immune dysfunction in FM is still unresolved. FM is often associated with autoimmune disorders. Immunofluorescent abnormalities in skin biopsies are an inconstant finding. Cytokine measurements have been unremarkable in published work by others, although my experience is somewhat different. Signs of immune activation are frequent. Elevation in levels of the IL-2 receptor, the soluble CD8 receptor, the HLA-DR receptor and numbers of CD3+, CD38+ cells are fairly common. Natural killer (NK) function is often reduced. Delayed-type hypersensitivity testing with the multitest-CMI system usually shows anergy or hypoergy. Abnormalities in 2,5A synthetase/RNase L have been described in primarily fibromyalgic patients receiving Ampligen. Immune substances such as IL-1 and TNF are involved in the maintenance of NREM sleep. Poly I:C, a compound closely related to Ampligen, has also been noted to stimulate NREM sleep. FM, like CFS (and it is often hard to distinguish between the two), sometimes begins with a flu-like illness and it is possible that a persistent state of immune activation is produced.

We have studied a group of patients with "primary fibromyalgia" from a brain function point of view. There were 12 patients who had few other symptoms besides the requisite 11/18 tender points, and no perceived cognitive dysfunction. My hypothesis was that they would have subclinical abnormalities of the electrophysiologic and neuropsychologic parameters that we measured in CFS. BEAM scans all showed temporal lobe dysfunction. An encoding difficulty, although to a modest degree, was found in all patients, arguing for the concept of a CNS lesion as a unifying characteristic.

The limbic system, as a regulator of autonomic function, could certainly produce hypoperfusion in muscle, just as it does in the brain in CFS. Our PET scan data show hypometabolism in the hippocampus, dorsolateral prefrontal cortex, and cingulate gyrus, as would be expected in CFS, but also often in the anterior cerebellum, posterior parietal lobe, superior colliculus, anterior caudate, and premotor cortex. The cerebellum regulates muscle tone via the gamma motoneurons and perhaps also has input to the Golgi tendon organs (not all tender points are in muscle). Although FM patients do not demonstrate hyperreflexia, and may not manifest muscle spasm (although some do), the fact that cyclobenzaprine (Flexeril) modulates the gamma motoneuron and is effective in FM suggests a possibility for dysfunction of this circuit. The midline cerebellum (vermis and fastigial nucleus) has been demonstrated to be part of a neural network with connections to the limbic system.[63] The fastigial nucleus is also involved in a primary vasodilator system linked to nitric oxide.[64] An abnormality in the premotor cortex, which is related to voluntary initiation of motor activity, is more difficult to explain. All that I could say would be that this region, involved with motor function, may be functioning abnormally, but the manner in which it would contribute to the pathogenesis of CFS/FM is unclear. FM patients, like those with IBS and panic disorder, are said to be more sensitive to pain and more vigilant about their bodily functions. All of these hypometabolic areas, with the exception of the anterior cerebellum, are projection areas of the dorsolateral prefrontal cortex.[65]

Lymphadenalgia

Painful lymph nodes are one of the diagnostic characteristics of CFS. This finding actually is not too common, and probably what were described by early investigators were actually the tender points of FM in sites near lymph nodes, or tender carotid bulbs as are seen in carotidynia. Lymph node enlargement is not frequently seen either, and little is known about the sensory innervation of lymph nodes. Sensory nerves are said to be associated with blood vessels. VIP and peptide histidine isoleucine regulate blood flow through lymphocytes but VIP probably is not involved in lymphadenalgia, since administration of a somatostatin analog, octreoide (Sandostatin), which tends to be a VIP antagonist, has no effect on lymphadenalgia.

Substance P/CGRP fibers may be lymph node afferents.[66] Nerves to lymph nodes come from both the vagus and the sympathetic ganglia, and the function of the autonomic nervous system can be modulated by descending input as has been discussed for other symptoms. In my experience, lymphadenalgia is most frequently encountered in the axillary region. One wonders whether this pain is actually from lymphatic tissue at all, since the primary human site of BAT is in the axillary regions, and I know of no specific difference in the role of axillary lymph nodes from those elsewhere in the body. A myofascial pain syndrome in the pectoralis muscle, common in CFS, can sometimes produce a medial axillary pain.

Premenstrual syndrome (PMS), also known as late luteal phase dysphoria (LLPD), is almost invariably present in CFS. If it did not exist before the onset of CFS it develops after the onset. Pre-existing PMS is greatly worsened. It seems rather obvious that PMS is caused by a dysregulation of receptors for ovarian steroids, and those in the limbic system are prime candidates. Many of the symptoms of PMS are also those of CFS, and limbic structures such as the amygdala are known to concentrate ovarian steroids. Estrogen and progesterone have genomic and non-genomic effects on cell function, the non-genomic ones having to do with alteration of membrane excitability.[67,68] There is an intricate relationship between GnRH, ovarian steroids, pituitary gonadotropins, endogenous opioids, prostaglandins, neurotransmitters, and IL-1.[69] Other cytokines have not been studied, to my knowledge. Estrogen and progesterone have immunomodulatory effects of their own, progesterone being generally immunosuppressive. Both estradiol and progesterone suppress the secretion of IL-1 from luteal phase macrophages. The immunosuppression of pregnancy is due, in part, to progesterone priming of pregnancy-sensitized lymphocytes so that suppressor-cell function can be induced by an as yet unnamed cytokine.[70] Although progesterone agonists may be successful in eliminating PMS symptoms, they may not act through anovulation, but rather by stimulating limbic-hypothalamic progesterone receptors. Metabolic products of progesterone, the neurosteroids, further open the chloride channel in the $GABA_A$ receptors. They have no "hormonal" effects, and longer-acting synthetic analogs may be useful in treating PMS. Neurosteroids are manufactured in the brain.[71]

It has been difficult to demonstrate a progesterone abnormality consistently in PMS, but the pulsatile nature of luteinizing hormone (LH) secretion may be dysregulated. The GnRH control over LH secretion is modulated in part by endogenous opioids. IL-1 may exert many of its limbic effects through endogenous opioids,[72] since some of its hypothalamic actions can be blocked by naloxone. If CFS is, in part, a disorder of cytokine dysregulation, IL-1 could be secreted by the hippocampus and affect the hypothalamus, or it could gain slow access from the periphery via the circumventricular organs: area postrema, organum vasculosum, choroid plexus (which also manufactures IL-1), pineal gland (perhaps not involved in PMS since melatonin biosynthesis is not abnormal in PMS), and median eminence. A bidirectional transport of IL-1 alpha across the blood-brain-barrier (BBB) has been demonstrated,[73] although this finding has not been confirmed by others. The hypothalamus had the highest entry rate. Activated T-lymphocytes may also cross the BBB and release IL-1 (and presumably other cytokines) into particular sites. The circumventricular organs may also function as neuronal transducers of circulating peripheral neuropeptides and cytokines, manufacturing them without allowing their ingress.[74]

IL-1 receptors are where one would expect them to be;[75] this localization has been questioned by some researchers who are unable to find them outside the hypothalamus and choroid plexus. They have been reported in the arcuate nucleus, periventricular and preoptic regions, retrochiasmatic area, central nucleus of the amygdala, periaqueductal gray, bed nucleus of the stria terminalis, midline thalamic nuclei, locus ceruleus, parabrachial nuclei, dorsal raphe nuclei, and the nucleus tractus solitarius. Other hypothalamic areas also have IL-1 receptors. Many of these areas are also quite estrogen-sensitive as well as progesterone-sensitive either with or without progesterone priming. Both recombinant human IL-1 alpha and IL-1 beta block the progesterone-induced LH surge and thus may alter the low frequency, high amplitude pattern of LH secretion seen in the luteal phase of women without PMS.[76] The effects of IL-1 on pituitary hormone release occur at concentrations within the range of IL-1 in serum, and IL-1 levels increase after ovulation. A direct stimulatory effect of IL-1 on adrenal glucocorticoid production has been demonstrated. One-third of patients with CFS, according to the work of Klimas et al., have quite elevated levels of IL-1 alpha mRNA.[77] CFS patients, however, do not have hypercortisolemia, and may be relatively resistant to ACTH stimulation. The mechanism for this resistance is perhaps due to decreased ACTH secretion, a result of central CRH underproduction, so that the adrenal cortex is not capable of responding to exogenous ACTH stimulation as it should. Levels of mRNA for other cytokines are being investigated in several laboratories. Serum cytokine measurements may be unreliable in CFS due to the presence of inhibitors.

No cytokine has been investigated as extensively as IL-1 for its CNS effects, but it is likely that other immune transmitters have an effect on ovarian steroid receptor sensitivity and on regulation of GnRH and gonadotropin secretion, as well as more general effects on limbic receptors of various sorts. Just as it is difficult to explain the symptoms of CFS without invoking limbic mechanisms, so is it puzzling to understand PMS.

Remembering that the limbic system amplifies and refines the control and function of the hypothalamus, just as the hypothalamus does for the brain stem, we can appreciate its role in PMS.[78] The limbic system permits primitive cognitive functions and primary emotions. The heteromodal and paralimbic areas amplify and regulate the control of the limbic system in a more complex and sophisticated manner, so that state variables (cognition and attitude) have more of an influence. Temporolimbic structures do not have their primary effect in the reverberating circuit proposed by Papez. This concept proposes that the "limbic" cortex, which "rims around" the medical aspect of the telencephalon is a largely self-contained functional system.[79] Rather, they directly innervate structures downstream in the neuraxis: the diencephalon, brain stem, and even the spinal cord. All of these structures have feedback or feedforward relationships with one another, but if the concept of limbic derangement of normal physiology were integrated into general medical thinking, many disorders (not just CFS, although CFS incorporates many of them) would be better understood.

CFS patients are often thirsty. The traditional regulators of thirst are osmoreceptors controlling release of vasopressin, and volume receptors which secrete atrial natriuretic peptide. CGRP (calcitonin gene-related peptide) has recently been added to the list as a promotor of venous capacitance. There is little evidence to suggest that these mechanisms are operative in CFS. Psychogenic polydipsia is sometimes seen. The most powerful stimulus to thirst is angiotensin II, and the receptors for this peptide in the brain may be dysregulated in CFS. Treatment with angiotensin-converting enzyme inhibitors is sometimes effective.[80] Nitric oxide acts as an inhibitory mechanism when thirst is stimulated by water deprivation or angiotensin II in the preoptic area.[81] If nitric oxide synthase is inhibited, psychogenic polydipsia could ensue. Sicca syndrome is frequently seen in the CFS patient. Sjogren antibodies are not present although enhancement of the salivary glands on MRI in CFS patients with positive antinuclear antibodies is rarely present. The Schirmer test is often positive. This deficit is probably due to dysfunctional autonomic control of tear and saliva secretion and waxes and wanes along with other symptoms. It could also be caused via descending pathways to brain stem parasympathetic nuclei.

CFS patients have several respiratory complaints. Air hunger, dyspnea at rest, and dyspnea on minimal exertion, sometimes thought to be asthma, are fairly common. Many have a history consistent with hyperventilation syndrome, and when asked to hyperventilate voluntarily in the office, reproduction of some symptoms may occur. The presence of hyperventilation syndrome is thought to mean that the patient has an anxiety disorder, or another diagnosis, "effort syndrome," which is conceptually related to neurasthenia. Most authorities do not address the reason why patients have these abnormalities, although central dysfunction of CO_2 or pH receptors has been suggested. The lowering of PCO_2 and raising of pH, however, is the opposite of what one sees in the provocation of panic attacks by CO_2 inhalation.

We have seen irregular respiratory rhythms in CFS patients who are maximally exercised, a finding which has never been described in anyone under these conditions.[82] We also see inappropriate hyperventilation at the onset of exercise, especially in CFS patients with FM. Irregular rhythms of this sort have been noted in patients with anxiety disorder at rest, but never while exercising. Maximal exertion typically abolishes this type of abnormality. These findings are one reason why we postulate a dysregulation in the central control of respiration. The most likely location for this disorder to occur, based on what has already been discussed, is the amygdala, although frontal lobe and paralimbic structures may also be involved.

The central nuclei of the amygdala have a massive projection to the pneumotaxic center in the pons. Single pulse stimulation of these amygdalar nuclei in monkeys causes an immediate switch to inspiration.[83] I can think of no other single reason to explain the respiratory abnormalities that we see in CFS other than this sort of amygdalar dysfunction. The limbic system has been shown to regulate automatic, but not voluntary, respiration.[84]

It would be possible to consider each and every symptom of CFS and its relationship to limbic neuroimmune function, but the story would begin to get redundant. However, I would like to consider four more symptoms:

1. Disorders of urinary urgency, frequency, and nocturia
2. Decreased libido
3. Disorders of temperature regulation and sensitivity to hot and cold ambient environments
4. Alcohol intolerance

These are so characteristic of CFS that an understanding of them may shed light on pathophysiology.

Detrusor dyssynergia is the most common urologic complaint, with interstitial cystitis being a somewhat distant second. Afferent and efferent fibers of the appropriate spinal segments are connected to the so-called micturition centers in the pontomesencephalic tegmentum. Afferent impulses to these centers come from the sacral cord. Descending fibers course through the reticulospinal tracts to the quaintly named "nucleus of Onuf," a densely packed group of somatomotor neurons in the anterior horns of sacral segments 1, 2, and 3. The micturition centers receive descending fibers from several limbic regions.

Frontal lobe incontinence may present in an incomplete form of frequency and urgency. Lesions in the anterior cingulate gyrus can cause these symptoms, and we frequently see such lesions on PET scan. A characteristic SPECT scan lesion in CFS is right dorsolateral prefrontal hypoperfusion. It would not be surprising if aberrations in mucosal immunity which could cause interstitial cystitis or recurrent urinary tract infections could be caused by dysregulation of the innervation of immunocytes in bladder epithelium.

Decreased libido is an almost universal complaint among CFS patients. Most biologic studies of libido have been done in women. It is difficult to find an animal model for what has been called hypoactive sexual desire disorder (HSD).[85] In subprimate mammals, sexual behavior is closely linked to estrous and the activating effect of estrogen. Some species may demonstrate an inhibiting effect of progesterone. The female is only sexually receptive and attractive to the male during estrous. Subhuman primates are sexually receptive throughout the menstrual cycle although more so at midcycle. Studies of normal women and those with HSD fail to reveal any cyclicity to sexual desire, and there are no hormonal differences between the two groups. An abnormality in gonadal steroid receptor regulation is a possibility in the HSD population, perhaps due to a dysregulation in the steroid environment of the brain in fetal life. Paralimbic inputs to relevant limbic structures could also be altered, since cognitive and attitudinal factors are so important in sexual arousal. Similar mechanisms could exist in the CFS patient, who differs from the HSD patient in that about one-third of the latter group has *never* been sexually aroused at all. A CFS deficiency in DHEA, an adrenal androgen, or its receptors could be related to decreased libido. Other androgenic neurosteroids could also be implicated.

Temperature regulation occurs, in part, in the anterior hypothalamus, where the "thermostat" is. This group of cells senses the temperature of the blood flowing through this region and adjusts the heat conservation and dissipation mechanisms accordingly. The most effective way the body has to eliminate heat is by perspiration, which involves the sympathetic and parasympathetic nervous system and cutaneous vasodilatation. Body temperature can be regulated by altering the hypothalamic "set point." Fever is probably caused by cytokines such as IL-1 which has a dense receptor population in the anterior hypothalamus. CFS patients are well known to have disorders of temperature regulation. Perhaps one-third have intermittent mild fevers. More commonly, subnormal temperatures are encountered, although patients may feel warm. Night sweats occur primarily in NREM sleep and may be related to the alpha-EEG abnormality and dysregulation of nocturnal IL-1 secretion. The perspiration that CFS patients report is not due to gonadal steroid insufficiency with elevated gonadotropic hormones, since estrogen replacement therapy is usually ineffective, and other signs of a menopausal syndrome are not present. Elevated levels of cytokines in the CFS patient may be responsible for raising the hypothalamic set point in some patients, but a more likely cause is a hypothalamic dysfunction in the autonomic integration required for the maintenance of body temperature. Supporting this hypothesis is the observation that alterations in temperature can increase CFS symptomatology. The most obvious example is in Raynaud's syndrome. A subpopulation of patients with fibromyalgia have increased density of platelet alpha-2 adrenergic receptors, which may predispose them to cold-induced and emotionally induced vasospasm.[86] Platelet adrenergic receptor status may mirror that of the brain adrenergic receptors. Thus it is likely that either alpha-2 adrenergic receptor density is altered in limbic structures, and/or that the regulation of expression of peripheral adrenergic receptors is deranged. Efferent pathways from the anterior hypothalamus to other limbic structures and to the periphery may be responsible for CFS relapse during hot or cold weather. The increased density of alpha-2 adrenergic receptors may be responsible for some of the pain in FM as well, since autonomic dysregulation of blood flow to muscles has been postulated as being contributory to FM, and sometimes regional sympathetic blockade relieves pain in FM. Clonidine often relieves CFS night sweats, probably by its action as a presynaptic alpha-2 agonist. Heat often exacerbates CFS symptoms, as it does to those of multiple sclerosis. Heat and humidity have been suggested as the precipitants of summer seasonal affective disorder.

The mechanism of the intoxicating effects of alcohol has still not been established as of this writing, but it is uncommon to interview a CFS patient who is not intolerant of alcohol. Intoxication may be produced by small amounts of alcohol previously well tolerated, alcohol may produce a dysphoric effect, hangovers may be severe, and/or an increase in CFS symptoms may occur after alcohol consumption. Intestinal candidiasis, a controversial entity, may cause some of its symptoms by production of ethanol and acetaldehyde and their effect on limbic structures.

Current thinking is that ethanol specifically and selectively affects the function of certain membrane-bound proteins, which include receptor-gated ion channels. $GABA_A$ and NMDA ion channels are prime candidates for this action. The $GABA_A$ receptor occurs in multiple receptor clones with different types of polypeptide subunits.[87] There are, for example, high concentrations of the alpha-2 and alpha-4 subunits in the hippocampus, with different cell types within the hippocampus having different proportions of alpha subunits. $GABA_A$ subunits are decreased in chronic ethanol users, and this feature may be involved in alcohol withdrawal. Ethanol stimulates chloride ion flux through the $GABA_A$ receptor-gated chloride channels. It is possible that $GABA_A$ receptor density could be altered in CFS or that the subunit composition of receptors in various sites could be altered. The general effects of GABA, an inhibitory neurotransmitter which is part of the macromolecular benzodiazepine receptor, are too complex to discuss here. It has been implicated in the pathogenesis of Huntington disease, Parkinsonism, epilepsy, schizophrenia, anxiety disorders, and tardive dyskinesia.

Ethanol is a potent inhibitor, at low concentrations, of the NMDA receptor-gated ion channel.[88] There may also be subtypes of the NMDA receptor, the channels of which are opened by glycine. Glycine reverses NMDA inhibition by ethanol in several brain regions. NMDA receptors are excitatory, and the subtype that is activated by glutamate is the most affected by ethanol. It would be congruent with other observations in CFS patients to hypothesize that glutamate-sensitive NMDA receptors are increased. Ethanol may also inhibit G proteins, as general anesthetics have been hypothesized to do.[89] G protein inhibition may be the reason why some CFS patients relapse after general anesthesia. If nitric oxide synthase levels are decreased in CFS, the effect of halothane anesthesia may be augmented, suggesting a role for nitric oxide in mediating consciousness.[90]

Most classical neurotransmitters are affected by ethanol, and one other finding is that catecholamine-aldehyde condensation products, thought to be how ethanol might intoxicate, are highly concentrated in the limbic system.[91] The opioid system, well represented in limbic structures, is also involved, as is the dopaminergic system, perhaps in the nucleus accumbens. Serotoninergic neurons are related to alcohol craving, with frequent reports of decreased desire for ethanol after fluoxetine or buspirone. As the mechanism of ethanol intoxication and withdrawal is better understood, so will our knowledge of the pathogenesis of CFS symptoms be enhanced.

OVERVIEW

In this chapter I have focused on the limbic etiology of several CFS symptoms. I have deliberately not emphasized infectious, immunologic, neuroendocrine, or peripheral metabolic factors. I have omitted a detailed discussion of neurotransmitter variables, since our knowledge of fluctuations in levels of these substances in limbic structures is rudimentary and could probably best be determined by permanent catheterization of limbic structures in primates. Functional brain imaging by SPECT and PET with receptor labeling is imminent and will enhance our understanding of this variable. Several points should be important in our future understanding of limbic encephalopathy in a dysregulated neuroimmune network:

1. The limbic system should be viewed as a higher order, sophisticated regulatory system responding to a wide variety of inputs. Cognitive, behavioral, and attitudinal changes can alter the state of limbic elements. This alteration can best be understood at present neuropathically by electrophysiologic measurements, but must also be mediated neurochemically. Diffuse projection systems such as exist for dopamine, norepinephrine, serotonin, and acetylcholine could be rapidly modulated in this manner, but take seconds to occur. Changes induced by amino acid transmitters such as glutamate and glycine are seen in microseconds, as are those mediated by G proteins, and perhaps these agents are more relevant to state changes. The concept of the regulatory limbic system is the most important one in this book.

2. The fact that autonomic transmission to a particular organ system can be regulated independently of the rest of the autonomic nervous system (ANS) is unfamiliar to many. The neurophysiology of such regulation is not understood at present, but can be experimentally demonstrated. This finding is particularly relevant when innervation of individual immunocytes or ganglia is considered.

3. There are undoubtedly multiple types of CFS. In the simplest division, there may be a discrimination of symptoms exacerbated by exercise (possibly from cytokine receptors), stress (possibly from limbic neurotransmitters), and intellectual effort (possibly from glutamatergic dysregulation of "fragile" neurons).[92,93] All may be mediated by IL-1, however. A causal typology is of value. Patients who have an acute "viral" type of onset probably have the best prognosis, although a recent prospective study of patients with infectious mononucleosis[94] revealed that a surprisingly high percentage went on to chronic illness, and investigation in a chronic

fatigue clinic indicated that those with an acute viral onset had the highest degree of psychopathology.[95] Many CFS patients with FM appear to have different neurochemistry and functional neuroanatomy than do CFS patients without FM. Dysregulation of the central neurogenic control of cerebral circulation is present in the majority of CFS patients, and may produce symptoms related to persistent regional ischemia.

4. Generation of CFS symptoms by dysregulation of cytokines is an attractive hypothesis. Many patients have elevated IL-2R levels, and elevated IL-2 and IL-1 levels have been reported.[96] It is difficult to measure cytokine levels. Cytokine mRNA, determined by PCR, should be more accurate. Limbic dysfunction could be produced by altered levels of cytokines made within the brain or peripherally, since peripheral cytokines may alter CNS cytokine levels via the circumventricular organs. Another likely possibility is that limbic cytokine receptors could be up- or down- regulated, so that normal cytokine levels could produce abnormal effects. IL-1 receptor expression can be upregulated in mouse pituitary tumor cells by CRH.[97] Could a deficiency of CRH downregulate them?

5. The notion that limbic dysfunction is the final common pathway for numerous potentially noxious insults helps one to understand the pathogenesis of numerous psychiatric, psychosomatic, and "organic" disorders. Although suggested by the Soviets and E. Fuller Torrey for many years, the viral role in psychiatric disorders is still poorly understood. One viral candidate is human foamy virus. Transgenic mice expressing the human foamy virus gene demonstrate reactive gliosis and neuronal degeneration which is most marked in the telencephalon and the CA3 hippocampal layer. No inflammation was seen in the brains of the animals, who also had a myopathy. If the psychoneuroimmunologic postulate that psychological influences can do most things that viruses can do is correct, then a virus may provide a bridge between the "psychological" and "organic." Other candidate viruses are that of Borna disease, recently identified by PCR,[98] HHV-6, intracisternal viruses, and enteroviruses, which are popular among British viral immunologists working in CFS.

Studies of the HIV-1-associated cognitive/motor complex have yielded hypotheses similar to those suggested here.[99] The HIV-1 envelope protein gp120 has been a favorite candidate for a neuro-toxic gene product. It can cause increases in intracellular calcium which can be blocked by calcium channel blockers, in concert with glutamate which binds to the NMDA receptor. Toxic effects of gp120 can be blocked in vitro by NMDA receptor antagonists as well as by peptide T, perhaps via its action as a VIP agonist.[100,101]

This concept is quite similar to that of cellular injury in cerebral ischemia developed by Choi.[102] The injury should be able to be antagonized by peptide T, which blocks gp120 receptor attachment. We are planning a double-blind study of this compound in CFS dementia.

HIV-1 infected macrophages have been found to secrete cytokines, and such compounds may have a mediating role in dementia. In CFS abnormal cytokine secretion by neurons or glial cells may occur, since viral infection of CNS macrophages has not been demonstrated.

6. A commonality to all neurasthenic syndromes may be a central deficiency of CRH secretion. Not only does decreased CRH cause central hypocortisolemia, but it also has numerous possible transmitter functions apart from its stimulatory effect on ACTH secretion. The best known is a facilitatory role in sympathetic nervous system function.[103] In this role it acts predominantly on limbic structures, but it is also present in cerebrospinal fluid and probably acts at the brain stem and spinal cord levels as well. Central administration of CRH causes increased motor activity, increased plasma levels of catecholamines and vasopressin, and an increase in the metabolic rate. Body temperature might be raised slightly, and CRH promotes brown fat thermogenesis. CRH receptors are also found on splenic macrophages, testis, pancreas, and adrenal medulla, suggesting multiple effects of this peptide. It would be rational to give exogenous vasopressin, perhaps in the form of DDAVP, to patients with neurasthenic syndromes, but my experience with this therapeutic modality has been generally disappointing. Treatment of CFS patients with corticosteroids has been similarly unhelpful. CRH is not yet on the market, and long acting forms of it are not available. Side effects of CRH appear to be minimal, with facial flushing occurring in about 30% of patients. A CRH antagonist, alpha-helical CRH, could have utility in the treatment of major depressive disorder or anxiety. Atypical depression may be characterized by low CRH levels.[104] Patients with CFS, as well as many

of those with atypical depression, have low levels of urinary cate-cholamine metabolites, probably an effect of decreased CRH levels. One study, suggesting that CFS patients were dysautonomic, re-ported elevated levels of plasma norepinephrine, however.[105]

It is likely that CRH is an important, perhaps the most important, neuropeptide involved in CFS. A decreased level of central CRH could upregulate CRH receptors and increase the opportunity for viral infection of a cell through this receptor. Such a genetic neuroen-docrine tendency could account for CFS occurring in certain person-ality types. A corollary to this hypothesis would be that lymphocytes of these patients would not secrete as much CRH in stress situations. Perhaps their CRH (and ACTH) receptors would be upregulated as well. Their IL-1 receptors might be downregulated, however.

7. Immune abnormalities in CFS are inconsistent. The work of Landay, Jessop, Estelle, and Levy[106] which demonstrates immune activation, particularly of the cytotoxic T lymphocytes, meshes nicely with the results of Klimas, who finds that there is a deficit in the function and number of suppressor-inducer T lymphocytes. Thus, one way to look at CFS is as an impairment of suppression of the immune response. This effect could be a result of a persistent viral infection, or a "hit-and-run" infection by an agent which would impair suppressor-inducer function, or both. Hypocortisole-mia has also been suggested as a cause of immune activation. Natu-ral killer cell number may be increased but function may be de-creased. The reasons for these findings are under investigation. Lymphocytes from CFS patients do not generate IL-2 and gamma interferon when stimulated, a result which distinguishes them from lymphocytes of patients with multiple sclerosis. Since there appears to be little or no CNS inflammatory response in CFS, one reason may be deficient production of gamma interferon, which induces expression of the class I MHC receptor. Cytotoxic T lymphocytes will not attack a cell which does not express this receptor, a mecha-nism demonstrated by Oldstone and colleagues[107] for persistence of lymphocytic choriomeningitis virus in neuronal cells. Perhaps this receptor is not expressed in virally mediated cases of CFS. The neural regulation of these functions is currently speculative at best. If processed viral antigen displayed on cell membranes contains self-antigen for certain individuals, lymphocytes may become sen-

sitized to this antigen and cause the mild autoimmune phenomena observed in numerous CFS patients. This attractive concept is not supported by the absence of inflammatory cells in cerebrospinal fluid of CFS patients. If one does assume immune activation is central to the pathogenesis of CFS then the superantigen concept should be considered.[108]

Lymphocytes can be stimulated in a rather non-specific manner if an antigen combines with a part of the regulatory T-cell receptor which is not in the recognition groove for processed antigen from antigen-presenting cells. Such antigens are called superantigens and can be encoded by retroviruses in mice. This non-specific activation has been implicated in the pathogenesis of multiple sclerosis and may account for elevated viral antibody titers seen in CFS, as well as in MS. The type of immune response might depend on what type of antigens are encoded by the retrovirus and how they bind to various sites on the T-cell receptor.

8. CFS is the result of an interplay of genetic, environmental, and infectious factors. Genetic factors may not just include variable expression of membrane receptors that allow CFS virus to enter, but also would relate to the interaction of cellular genes with CFS virus(es) and other agents which could transactivate them. HLADR4 receptor expression appears to be increased in CFS patients in my patient population, but not in another.[109] If patients who are depressed, anxious, or borderline are more likely to develop CFS, this tendency may be attributable to a genetic or acquired limbic dysfunction. Environmental factors could include exposure to toxic agents such as hydrocarbons, insecticides, and tung oil, a phorbol ester. Hydrocarbons have been shown to produce a limbic encephalopathy on PET scan. I prefer to view genetic susceptibility in CFS as being on a continuum. Someone who was extremely susceptible could have CFS incited by a minute amount of a triggering agent. Some patients relate that they have always felt like they have had CFS. It is difficult to know whether they were born with it or contracted it early in childhood. These patients are more likely to have family histories of CFS or autoimmune disorders. Other patients seem to require prolonged, intense exposure to a triggering agent. Most spouses of CFS patients do not get CFS, but a few of them do. Their symptoms usually begin several years after the

partner's. This delayed or latent period before signs of infection is characteristic of retroviruses. Susceptibility to toxic agents may also be genetically determined. Tung oil and hydrocarbons may be the main offenders.

9. IL-1, IL-6, and probably other cytokines stimulate CRH secretion. Protein kinase C and protein kinase A-dependent pathways are involved in the response of CRH to IL-1 beta.[110] Antagonists to IL-1, which are endogenous because mRNA for these antagonists has been detected in the hippocampus, hypothalamus, and cerebellum, could regulate IL-1 effect and also CRH secretion, at least to an extent. Perhaps a situation exists in CFS in which IL-1 antagonist is made in excess, accounting for decreased CRH levels, thus exemplifying an immune-neuroendocrine link. The central stress response could be initiated by IL-1 beta and dynamically modulated by various antagonists. Using this model for CFS, symptoms could be caused by excess or inadequate IL-1 beta effect, depending upon the concentrations of the various antagonists. Decreased levels of limbic eicosanoids are another possibility, since these mediate many IL-1 CNS actions. Neurotoxic gene products could alter expression of the IL-1 receptor on CRH- or ACTH-secreting cells, or impair translocation of the receptor or its secondary messengers. Nuclear or transcriptional events for CRH or ACTH are less likely to be altered, since the gene product would not be likely to have the same effect in both types of cells.

10. Another example of an immune-neuroendocrine link is the effect of Ampligen, a mismatched, double-stranded RNA related to Poly I:Poly C. This compound has been shown to have antiviral and immunomodulatory properties in a multicenter, double-blind experiment in patients with CFS. Researchers believe its effect is mediated through activity of the antiviral pathway of 2,5A synthetase/RNase L, which is increased in some patients with CFS. Patients have had marked increases in energy and cognitive function and a reduction in mood disorders while on this drug. The 2,5A pathway consumes ATP, so that less ATP is available for energy metabolism and also for stimulating ATP-activated channels found in muscle cells, neurons in the dorsal horn, and a small subset of cultured hippocampal neurons.[111] These channels are controlled by P_2 purinergic receptors.

REFERENCES

1. Layzer RB. How muscles use fuel. *N Engl J Med* 324(6): 411-412,1991.
2. Cheney P. Personal communication.
3. Karpati G. Presented at: Workshop on research directions for myalgic encephalomyelitis/chronic fatigue syndrome, Vancouver, Canada, May 11, 1991.
4. Simon HB. Exercise and human immune function. In: Ader R, Felten DF, Cohen N (eds.). Psychoneuroimmunology, second edition, San Diego: Academic Press, 1991.
5. Mena I. Presented at: Chronic Fatigue Syndrome and the Brain, Bel Air, CA, April 25,1992.
6. Ellison MD, Krieg RJ, Merchant RE. Cerebral vasomotor responses after recombinant interleukin-2 infusion. *Cancer Res* 50(14): 4377-4381, 1990.
7. Licinio J, Wong M-L, Gold PW. Localization of interleukin-1 receptor antagonist mRNA in rat brain. *Endocrinology* 129(1):562-564,1991.
8. Wu KK. Endothelial cells in hemostasis, thrombosis, and inflammation. *Hospital Practice* 27(4):145-168, 1992.
9. de Souza EB. Personal communication.
10. Kalkman HO, Fozard JR. 5HT receptor subtypes and their role in disease. *Curr Opinion Neurol Neurosurg* 4:560-565, 1991.
11. Raszkiewicz JL, Linville DG, Kerwin JF, Wagenaar F, Americ SP. Nitric oxide synthase is critical in mediating basal forebrain regulation of cortical cerebral circulation. *J Neurosci Res* 33:129-135, 1992.
12. Wilkins RH. Cerebral vasospasm: prevention and treatment. In: *Cerebral Blood Flow: Physiologic and Clinical Aspects.* Ed: Wood JH. New York, McGraw-Hill, 1987.
13. Takamatsu Y, Yamamoto H, Ogunremi OO, Matsuzaki I, Moroji T. The effects of corticotropin-releasing hormone on peptidergic neurons in the rat forebrain. *Neuropeptides* 20:255-265, 1991.
14. Weiss JM, Sundar SK, Becker KJ, Cierpial MA. Behavioral and neural influences on cellular immune responses: effects of stress and interleukin-1. *J. Clin Psychiatry* 50(5) (suppl): 43-52, 1989.
15. Saperstein A, Brand H, Audhya T, Nabriski D, Hutchinson B, Rosenzweig S, Hollander CS. Interleukin-1 beta mediates stress-induced immunosuppression via corticotropin-releasing factor. *Endocrinology* 130(1):152-158, 1992.
16. Moldofsky H. Non-restorative sleep and symptoms after afebrile illness in patients with fibrositis and chronic fatigue syndrome. *J Rheumatol* (suppl.) 19:150-153, 1989.
17. Reynolds WJ, Moldofsky H, Saskin P, Lue FA. The effects of cyclobenzaprine on sleep physiology and symptoms in patients with fibromyalgia. *J Rheumatol* 18(3): 452-454, 1991.
18. Bennett RM, Clark SR, Campbell SM, Burckhardt CS. Low somatomedin-C levels in fibromyalgia (poster). Presented at American College of Rheumatology, 55th annual scientific meeting, Boston, November 17-21, 1991.

19. Sandman, CA, Barron JL, Nackoul K, Goldstein J, Fidler F, Memory deficits associated with chronic fatigue immune dysfunction syndrome (CFIDS). *Biol Psychiatry* (in press), 1993.

20. Olney JW. Excitatory amino acids and neuropsychiatric disorders. *Biol Psychiatry* 26:505-525, 1989.

21. Kandel ER, Hawkins RD. The biological basis of learning and individuality. *Sci American* 267(3): 79-86, 1992.

22. Izquierdo I. Role of NMDA receptors in memory. *Trends Pharmacol Sci* 12:128-129, 1991.

23. Izquierdo I, Medina JH. GABA$_A$, receptor modulation of memory: the role of endogenous benzodiazepines. *Trends Pharmacol Sci* 12:260-265, 1991.

24. Sandman C. Chronic fatigue syndrome dementia. Presented at: Chronic Fatigue Syndrome and the Brain, Bel Air, CA, April 25, 1992.

25. Fuster JM. *The Prefrontal Cortex: Anatomy, Physiology and Neuropsychology of the Frontal Lobe,* second edition. New York, Raven Press, 1989.

26. Goldberg M. Personal communication, 1992.

27. Sadun A. Presented at: Chronic Fatigue Syndrome and the Brain, Bel Air, CA April 24-26,1992.

28. Hoyenga KB, Hoyenga KT. *Psychobiology: The Neuron and Behavior.* Pacific Grove, CA, Brooks/Cole, 1988.

29. Yunus MB. Fibromyalgia: a dysfunctional syndrome with chronic pain. *Adv Pain Res Ther* 20:133-140, 1992.

30. Gabbard GO. Psychodynamic psychiatry in the "Decade of the Brain." *Am J Psychiatry* 149(8): 991-998, 1992.

31. Russell IJ, Russell SJ, Cuevas R, Michalek J. Early life traumas and confiding in fibromyalgia syndrome (FS). *Arth Rheum* 35(4): S349, 1992.

32. Kranzler HR, Manu P, Hesselbrock VM, Love TJ, Matthews DA. Substance use disorders in patients with chronic fatigue. *Hosp Community Psychiatry* 42(9): 924-928,1991.

33. Kusher MG, Beitman BD. Panic attacks without fear: an overview. *Behav Res Ther* 28(6): 469-479, 1990.

34. Russell JL, Kushner MG, Beitman BD, Bartels KM. Nonfearful panic disorder in neurology patients validated by lactate challenge. *Am J Psychiatry* 148(3): 361-364, 1991.

35. Gorman JM, Liebowitz MR, Figer AJ, Stein J. A neuroanatomical basis for panic disorder. *Am J Psychiatry* 146(2): 148-161,1989.

36. Reiman EM, Fosselman MJ, Fox PT, Raichle ME. Neuroanatomical correlates of anticipatory anxiety. *Science* 243:1071-1073, 1989.

37. Drevets WC, Videen TO, MacLeod AH, Haller JW, Raichle ME. PET images of blood flow changes during anxiety: correction. *Science* 256:1696, 1992.

38. Weinberger DR, Berman KF, Suddath R, Fuller-Torrey E. Evidence of dysfunction of a prefrontal limbic network in schizophrenia: a magnetic resonance imaging and regional cerebral blood flow study of discordant monozygotic twins. *Am J Psychiatry* 149(7): 890-897, 1992.

39. Cooper JR, Bloom FE, Roth R. *The Biochemical Basis of Neuropharmacology,* sixth edition. New York, Oxford University Press, 1991.

40. Wood PL, Rao TS. Morphine stimulation of mesolimbic and mesocortical but not nigrostriatal dopamine release in the rat are reflected by changes in 3-methoxytyramine levels. *Neuropharmacology* 30(4):399-401, 1991.

41. Guilleminault C. Idiopathic central nervous system hypersomnia. In: Kryger MH, Roth T, Dement WC, *Principles and Practice of Sleep Medicine.* Philadelphia, Saunders, 1989.

42. Rusak B. The mammalian circadian system: models and physiology. *J Biol Rhythms* 4(2): 121-134,1989.

43. Stumpf WE, Privette TH. Light, vitamin D, and psychiatry: role of 1,25 dihydrovitamin D (soltriol) in etiology and therapy of affective disorder and other mental processes. *Psychopharmacology* 97:285-294, 1989.

44. Jones BE. Basic mechanisms of sleep-wake states. In: Kryger MH, Roth T, Dement WC. *Principles and Practice of Sleep Medicine.* Philadelphia, Saunders, 1989.

45. Sandyk R. Alpha rhythm and the pineal gland. *Intern J Neuroscience* 63:221-227, 1992.

46. Katon WH. Panic Disorder in the Medical Setting. Rockville, US Department of Health and Human Services, 1989.

47. Allen GV, Saper CB, Hurley KM, Cechetto DF. Organization of visceral and limbic connections in the insular cortex of the rat. *J Comp Neurol* 311:1-16, 1991.

48. Nilsson C, Lindvall-Axelsson M, Owman C. Neuroendocrine regulatory mechanisms in the choroid plexus-cerebrospinal fluid system. *Brain Res Rev* 17:109-138, 1992.

49. Sadun A. Presented at: Chronic Fatigue Syndrome and the Brain, Bel Air, CA April 24-26, 1992.

50. Wada Y, Hasegawa H, Nakamura M, Yamaguchi N. Serotoninergic inhibition of limbic and thalamic seizures in cats. *Neuropsychobiology* 25:87-90, 1992.

51. Post RM, Rubinow DR, Ballenger JC. Conditioning and sensitization in the longitudinal course of affective illness. *Br J Psychiatry* 149:191-201, 1986.

52. Goetzl EJ, Turck CW, Sreedharan SP. Production and reception of neuropeptide by cells of the immune system. In: Ader R, Felten DF, Cohen N (eds.). *Psychoneuroimmunology,* second edition. San Diego, Academic Press, 1991.

53. Shipley M. Transport of molecules from nose to brain: Transneuronal antegrade and retrograde labeling in the rat olfactory system by wheat germ agglutinin-horseradish peroxidase applied to the nasal epithelium. *Brain Res Bull* 15:129-142, 1985.

54. Himms-Hagen J. Neural control of brown adipose tissue thermogenesis, hypertrophy, and atrophy. *Prog Neuroendocrinol* 12(1): 38-93, 1991.

55. Ludwig H, Bade L, Gostony G. Borna disease: a persistent virus infection of the central nervous system. *Prog Med Virol* 34:107-151,1988.

56. Ricaurte GA, Molliver ME, Martello MB, Katz JL, Wilson MA, Martello AL. D-fenfluramine neurotoxicity in brain of non-human primates. *Lancet* 338: 1487, 1991.

57. Mathias JR. Personal communication, 1992.

58. Mathias JR, Ferguson KL, Clench MH. Debilitating "functional" bowel disease controlled by leuprolide acetate, gonadotropin-releasing hormone (GnRH) analog. *Dig Dis Sci* 34(5): 761-766, 1989.

59. Bothe K, Aguzzil A, Lassman H, Rethwilm A, Horak I. Progressive encephalopathy and myopathy in transgenic mice expressing human foamy virus genes. *Science* 253:555-557, 1991.

60. Blundell J. Pharmacological approaches to appetite suppression. *Trends Pharmacol Sci* 12(4):147-157, 1991.

61. Geracioti TD, Orth DN, Ekhator NN, Blumenkopf B, Loosen PT. Serial cerebrospinal fluid cortico-tropin releasing hormone concentrations in healthy and depressed humans. *J Clin Endocrinol Metab* 74(6):1325-1330, 1992.

62. Hedges HH. The elimination diet as a diagnostic tool. *Am Fam Physician* 46(5): 775-865, 1992.

63. Bench CJ, Friston KJ, Brown RG, Scott LC, Frackowiak RSJ, Dolan RJ. The anatomy of melancholia-focal abnormalities of cerebral blood flow in major depression. *J Clin Endocrinol Metab* 74(6):1325-1330, 1992.

64. Iadecola C. EDRF participates in the neocortical vasodilation elicited by stimulation of the fastigial nucleus. *Soc Neurosci Abstr* 17:6-9, 1991.

65. Goldman-Rakic PS. Prefrontal cortical dysfunction in schizophrenia: the relevance of the working memory. In: Carrol BJ, Barnett JE (eds.). *Psychology and the Brain*. New York, Raven Press, 1991.

66. Felten SY, Felten DL. Innervation of lymphoid tissue. In: Ader R, Felten DF, Cohen N (eds). *Psychoneuroimmunology,* second edition. San Diego: Academic Press, 1991.

67. McEwen BS. Non-genomic and genomic effects of steroids on neural activity. *Trends Pharmacol Sci* 12:141-147, 1991.

68. Delville Y. Progesterone facilitated sexual receptivity: a review of arguments supporting a nongenomic mechanism. *Neurosci Biobehav Rev* 15: 407-414, 1991.

69. Plata-Salaman CR. Immunoregulators in the nervous system. *Neurosci Biobehav Rev.* 13: 185-215, 1991.

70. Szekeres-Bartho J, Autran B, Debre P, Andreu G, Denver L, Chaouat G. Immunoregulatory effects of a suppressor factor from healthy pregnant women's lymphocytes after progesterone induction. *Cell Immunol* 122(2): 281-294,1989.

71. Deutsch SI, Mastropaolo J, Hitri A. GABA-active steroids: endogenous modulators of GABA-gated chloride ion conductance. *Clin Neuropharmacol* 15(5): 352-364, 1992.

72. Fagarasan MO, Arora PH, Axelrod J. Interleukin-1 potentiation of beta-endorphin secretion and the dynamics of interleukin-1 internalization in pituitary cells. *Drug Neuropsycho Biol Psychiatry* 15: 551-560, 1991.

73. Banks WA, Kastin AJ, Dorham DA. Bidirectional transport of interleukin-1 alpha across the blood-brain barrier. *Brain Res Bull* 23: 433-437, 1989.

74. Saper CB. Neurologic origin of fever. Presented at: The Seminar in Behavioral Neuroimmunology, UCLA School of Medicine, October 20, 1992.

75. Rothwell NJ. Functions and mechanisms of interleukin-I in the brain. *Trends Pharmacol Sci* 12(11): 430-436, 1991.

76. Facchinetti F, Genazzani AD, Martignoni E, Fioroni L, Sances G, Genazzani AR. Neuroendocrine correlates of premenstrual syndrome: changes in the pulsatile pattern of plasma LH. *Psychoneuroendocrinology* 15(4): 269-277, 1990.

77. Klimas N, Fletcher MA, Patarca R. Progress report. CFIDS Chronicle, 9-10, Fall 1991.

78. Gitlin MJ, Pasnau RO. Psychiatric syndromes linked to reproductive function in women: a review of current knowledge. *Amer J Psychiatry* 146(11): 1413-1421, 1989.

79. Papez JW. A proposed mechanism of emotion. *Arch Neurol Psychiatry* (Chicago) 38:725-743, 1937.

80. Goldstein JA. Captopril in the treatment of psychogenic polydipsia. *J Clin Psychiatry* 47(2): 99, 1986.

81. Calapai G, Squadrito F, Altavilla D, Zingarelli B, Campo GM, Cilia M, Caputi AP. Evidence that nitric oxide modulates drinking behavior. *Neuropharmacology* 31(8): 761-764, 1992.

82. Daly J. Presented at: Chronic Fatigue Syndrome and the Brain, Bel Air, CA, April 24-26, 1992.

83. Harper RM. Neurophysiology of sleep. In: Hypoxia, exercise and altitude: proceedings of the Third Banff International Hypoxia Symposium. New York: Alan R Liss, 65-73, 1991.

84. Munschauer FE, Mador MJ, Ahuja A, Jacobs L. Selective paralysis of voluntary but not limbically influenced automatic respiration. *Arch Neurol* 48:1190-1192, 1991.

85. Schreiner-Engel P, Schiavi RC, White D, Ghizzani A. Low sexual desire in women: The role of reproductive hormones. *Hormones and Behavior* 23: 221-234, 1989.

86. Bennett RM, Clark SR, Campbell CS, Ingram SB, Burckhardt CS, Nelson DL, Porter JM. Symptoms of Raynaud's syndrome in patients with fibromyalgia: a study using the Nielsen test, digital photoplethysmography, and measurements of platelet alpha-2 adrenegic receptors. *Arth Rheum* 34(3): 264-269, 1991.

87. Hanley JM, Johnstone GAR. Vintage amino acid meeting describes new tools for amino acid research, subtypes of metabotropic receptors. *Trends Pharmacol Sci* 12: 357-359, 1991.

88. Lovinger DM, White G, Weight FF. Ethanol inhibits NMDA-activated current in hippocampal neurons. *Science* 243: 1721-1724, 1989.

89. Anthony BL, Dennison RL, Aronstam RS. Disruption of muscarinic receptor G protein coupling is a general property of liquid volatile anesthetics. *Neurosci Lett* 99: 191-196, 1989.

90. Johns RA, Moscicki JC, Difazio CA. Nitric oxide synthase inhibitor dose-dependently and reversibly reduces the threshold for halothane anesthesia–a role for nitric oxide in mediating consciousness. *Anesthesiol* 77(4): 779-784, 1992.

91. Devenport LD, Hale RL. Contributions of hippocampus and neocortex to the expression of ethanol effects. *Psychopharmacology* 99:337-344, 1989.

92. Post RM. Transduction of psychosocial stress into the neurobiology of recurrent affective disorder. *Am J Psychiatry* 149(8):999-1010, 1992.

93. Rose SPR. How chicks make memories: the cellular cascade from c-fos to dendritic remodeling. *Trends Neurosci* 14: 390-397, 1991.

94. Lambore S, McSherry J, Kraus AS. Acute and chronic symptoms of mononucleosis. *J Family Practice* 33(1): 33-37, 1991.

95. Katon WJ, Buchwald DS, Simon GE, Russo JE, Mease PJ. Psychiatric illness in patients with chronic fatigue and those with rheumatoid arthritis. *J Gen Int Med* 6:277-285, 1991.

96. Hader N, Rimon D, Kinarty A, Lahat N. Altered interleukin-2 secretion in patients with primary fibromyalgia syndrome. *Arth Rheum* 34(7):866-871, 1991.

97. Webster EC, Tracey DE, DeSouza EB. Upregulation of interleukin-1 receptors in mouse AtT-20 pituitary tumor cells following treatment with corticotropin-releasing factor. *Endocrinology* 129(5): 2796-2798, 1991.

98. de La Torre JC, Carbone KM, Lipkin WI. Molecular characterization of the Borna disease agent. *Virology* 179(2):853-856, 1990.

99. Sharer LR. Pathology of HIV-1 infection of the central nervous system: a review. *J Neuropath Exp Neurol* 51(1):3-11, 1992.

100. Brenneman D. Neuroimmune interactions: implications for neuro-AIDS and neurodevelopment. Presented at: The Seminar in Behavioral Neuroimmunology, Los Angeles, UCLA School of Medicine, November 2, 1992.

101. Buzy J, Brenneman DE, Pert CB, Martin A, Salazar A, Ruff MR. Potent gp 120-like neurotoxic activity in the cerebrospinal fluid of HIV-infected individuals is blocked by peptide T. *Brain Res* 598:10:18, 1992.

102. Zivin JA, Choi DW. Stroke therapy. *Sci American* 265(1):56-65, 1991.

103. McCubbin JA, Kaufmann PG, Nemeroff CB. *Stress, neuropeptides, and systemic disease.* San Diego, Academic Press, 1991.

104. Demitrack MA, Greden JF. Chronic fatigue syndrome: The need for an integrative approach (editorial). *Biol Psychiatry* 30:747-752, 1991.

105. Levine S, Trestman R, Halper J, Cunningham-Rundles C. Plasma catecholamine levels in patients with chronic fatigue syndrome. Presented at: annual meeting, American Psychiatric Association, May 1990.

106. Landay AL, Jessop C, Lennette ET, Levy JA. Chronic fatigue syndrome: clinical condition associated with immune activation. *Lancet* 338:707-712, 1991.

107. Joly E, Mucke L, Oldstone MBA. Viral persistence in neurons explained by lack of major histocompatibility class I expression. *Science* 253:1283-1285, 1991.

108. Rudge P. Does a retrovirally encoded superantigen cause multiple sclerosis? *Neurol Neurosurg Psychiatry* 853-855, 1992.

109. Middleton D, Savage DA, Smith DG. No association of HLA class II antigens in chronic fatigue syndrome. *Dis Markers* 9:47-49, 1991.

110. Hu S-B, Tannahill LA, Lightman SL. Interleukin-1 beta increases corticotropin-releasing factor-41 release from cultured hypothalamic cells through protein kinase C and cAMP-dependent protein kinase pathways. *J Neuroimmunol* 40: 49-56, 1992.

111. O'Connor SE, Dainty IA, Leff P. Further subclassification of ATP receptors based on agonist studies. *Trends Pharmacol Sci* 12:137-141, 1991.

Diagnosis of Chronic Fatigue Syndrome

SUMMARY. The ambiguity of CFS diagnosis induced the convening of workshops to propose specific diagnostic criteria. An emphasis on the symptomatic overlap with the fibromyalgia syndrome (FMS) is discussed. Disorders associated with CFS include herpes simplex (both oral and genital), herpes zoster, psoriasis, urticaria, and atopic dermatitis. Another symptom is severe headaches, which are usually tension-type but may also be migrainous or related to benign intracranial hypertension. Cardiac complaints include supraventricular tachycardia and mitral valve prolapse. Abdominal symptoms are common, and many are caused by specific trigger points. Pelvic disease, especially endometriosis, adnexal masses, and polycystic ovarian syndrome, occur with greater frequency in CFS patients. The number of musculoskeletal abnormalities related to fibromyalgia is enormous. The lab tests necessary to rule out chronically fatiguing illnesses are discussed. Brain functional imaging is particularly useful, especially SPECT, but also PET and BEAM. It would be difficult to explain the entire constellation of CFS symptoms except by a model of limbic dysfunction or encephalopathy.

At first, the diagnosis of CFS appears to be insurmountably difficult. Fatigue can be caused by so many different disorders. After the first fifty patients or so are seen diagnosis seems easy, but it is not. A recent study of 200 patients with the chief complaint of "fatigue" revealed a physical illness in only ten of them.[1] Most fatigued patients have normal workups and it seems that the symptom profile of CFS is fairly distinctive, particularly if prolonged fatigue after

---

[DocuSerial™ co-indexing entry]

"Diagnosis of Chronic Fatigue Syndrome," Goldstein, J.A. Published in *Haworth Library of the Medical Neurobiology of Somatic Disorders* (The Haworth Medical Press), Volume 1, 1993 and *Chronic Fatigue Syndromes: The Limbic Hypothesis,* Goldstein, J.A., The Haworth Medical Press, 1993.

exercise, cognitive impairment, and recurrent flu-like illnesses with sore throat are noted. The presence of fibromyalgia tender points is always helpful in making an assessment. The reliability of the diagnosis is also enhanced if the initial symptoms developed rapidly in the context of a flu-like illness, and if premorbid nasal allergy was present.

Ambiguity in the diagnosis arises if the onset of the illness was gradual, if there are no flu-like symptoms, no fibromyalgia tender points, and if there is a history of psychiatric disorder antedating the illness. Patients from extremely dysfunctional families where there was child abuse are most difficult to diagnose since these individuals are prone to develop somatization disorder.

NIH RECOMMENDATIONS

A workshop was held at the National Institutes of Health in 1991 to refine the diagnostic criteria for CFS.[2] Patients with psychosis, substance abuse, and post-infectious fatigue with a definite etiology and an ongoing process were excluded from being diagnosed as having chronic fatigue syndrome. Fibromyalgia, post-infectious fatigue from an illness that had been adequately treated or should have resolved were included. Depression in the context of CFS was no longer exclusionary; it was suggested that note be made of whether it occurred concurrently with CFS, existed previously, or had resolved. Those diagnosed as having a somatization disorder were included, although it was not made explicit how these patients should be distinguished from those with CFS.

The following clinical evaluation was suggested:

1. Minimum laboratory tests. Those listed were CBC with differential, ESR, chemistry panel, TSH, and ANA and RF in those with myalgias. Ferritin levels and HIV testing were not included.
2. Screening for psychiatric distress done with a standard instrument. One structured interview was suggested, such as the Diagnostic Interview Schedule (DIS).
3. Tender points exam. This evaluation should minimize the symptoms of lymphadenalgia, which was probably confirmed by

palpation of unrecognized tender points. Lymphadenopathy is rather uncommon in my experience.
4. Serial examinations for emergence of other diagnoses, e.g., systemic lupus erythematosus or multiple sclerosis.

The group did not believe any laboratory tests are of value in confirming the diagnosis of CFS although appropriate lab tests were suggested to rule out other diagnoses. Tests regarded as experimental were immunologic and virologic tests, brain scans of all sorts, and neuroendocrine tests. Neuropsychological tests were not discussed and no mention was made of the cognitive impairment experienced by most CFS patients. The indications for polysomnography in this patient group were not considered. It was noted that objective measurements to assess CFS severity have not been validated.

The workshop participants concluded that CFS is not a homogeneous entity and that there is overlap with fibromyalgia and nonpsychotic depression, but that lab results from all groups are indistinguishable. Self-report was thought to be the best method of assessing illness severity. Standardization of assessment techniques including stratification of patients as to whether fibromyalgia, depression, criteria for somatization, and post-infectious fatigue were present were thought to be important. No mention was made of the hyperventilation provocation test.

As in previous efforts by such committees, the conclusions were extremely conservative and did not address important issues. CFS was still appropriately regarded as a syndrome, but no suggestion about etiology was even attempted. This deficiency reflects the division of opinion among those studying the illness. *There was no discussion of abnormalities in brain function being an aspect of CFS.* This omission was inexplicable to those of us who regard CFS as having important, if not primary, neurologic components. That these NIH recommendations may have become obsolete even before they were disseminated is suggested by the publication of experiments showing a specific kind of immune activation in CFS[3] and symptomatic and laboratory improvement in CFS with the immunomodulatory and antiviral drug Ampligen.[4] Even though psychological test results and brain imaging findings have been reported at meetings, none of the investigators who are involved in such work were invited to the workshop. The suggestions of this panel were similar to recommendations generated by a panel in Great Britain the previous year and published in the *Journal of the Royal Society of Medicine.*[5] The major addition of the NIH meeting was the mention of fibromyalgia.

CLINICAL SYMPTOMS

When I examine a patient suspected of having CFS, the presence of 11 out of 18 fibromyalgia tender points, with no tenderness at neutral points, is the only reliable physical sign and occurs in about two-thirds of this population. I feel much more confident about making the CFS diagnosis if the fibromyalgia tender points are present. Fibromyalgia may also be related to other conditions, primarily rheumatologic, but is also associated with infections, particularly viral. Bacterial, parasitic, and especially borrelia infections should also be considered. Fibromyalgia also may be seen in hypothyroidism. It can be distinguished without much difficulty from myofascial pain syndrome, which is local or regional, as well as from inflammatory and metabolic myopathies. Trigger points and fibromyalgia tender points may be activated by autonomic dysfunction causing decreased muscle blood flow. Raynaud's phenomenon is often associated with CFS/FM and can further reduce diagnostic ambiguity. (This physical sign was also not mentioned in either the NIH or British conference.) Positive Romberg tests, abnormal Hallpike maneuvers, and bilateral lower quadrant tenderness, either related to irritable bowel syndrome, pelvic disorders (especially endometriosis), or abdominal wall myofascial pain are commonly encountered. A frequent cause of pelvic pain in this population is pelvic floor tension myalgia, especially of the pyriform muscle. Palpation of the muscles associated with temporomandibular pain and dysfunction syndrome will frequently reveal tenderness, and this patient group should be investigated for bruxism.

Associated illnesses are extremely common, and virtually all of them could be caused by limbic encephalopathy. Let us consider some of them.

The major skin disorder is herpes simplex, both oral and genital. Herpes zoster is also fairly common. Psoriasis, urticaria, and atopic dermatitis are seen more often than in the general population and diffuse alopecia is seen more frequently than all of these conditions put together. Some of my patients have had to buy wigs. Minoxidil lotion may be of benefit. An inflammatory obliteration of fingerprints, as described by Cheney, occasionally occurs. The alopecia may sometimes be related to adrenal androgens and may be treated with low dose dexamethasone.

Severe headaches are quite common. These are usually of the tension-type, but can also be migrainous, related to TMPDS, or possibly to benign intracranial hypertension. I have seen only one CFS patient with cluster headache. Particularly in the CFS patient with a history of headache after a motor vehicle accident, myofascial trigger points in the head and neck should be examined.

Ocular complaints are common, but physical exam is usually negative except if one uses Frenzel glasses to look for nystagmus. Conjunctival injection and blepharitis are usually associated with nasal allergy. Schirmer tests are often positive. Some of these symptoms, including blurred vision, may be associated with sternomastoid trigger points in the sternal division. Although uncommon in CFS, these trigger points should be examined and treated if present.

The major otologic finding relates to TMPDS causing otalgia. Palpation of the medial pterygoid and superior masseter muscles will help to make the diagnosis. Evaluation of vertigo, tinnitus, and auditory discrimination disorders, common in CFS, has been previously discussed, although trigger points in the clavicular division of the sternomastoid can disturb proprioception and cause postural dizziness. Tinnitus can be caused by trigger points in the superior masseter.

Local nasal problems include allergic rhinitis or perennial rhinitis, intolerance of odors or fumes, and alteration in the sense of smell or taste. Rhinitis is extremely common and should not always be treated symptomatically. I order CT scans of the sinuses more frequently now in the fatigued patient with rhinitis; they are much more accurate than sinus X rays for diagnosing occult sinusitis. Many CFS symptoms, especially fatigue, will often improve when sinusitis is diagnosed and treated. On the other hand, numerous patients have had surgical procedures which have benefitted them transiently, if at all. Patients with environmental illnesses sometimes describe a generalization of their intolerances. Could this be due to kindling in the pyriform cortex?

While sore throat is quite common, pharyngitis is not. A common cause of throat (and ear) stuffiness in CFS is a trigger point in the medial pterygoid muscle, medial to the mandibular ramus and lateral to the last molar tooth. Patients will often have associated tenderness of the masseter and lateral pterygoid, but only the medial pterygoid refers pain to the tongue, pharynx, and hard palate. Sore throat has been experienced during the aura of limbic epilepsy.[6] Ear stuffiness occurs if spasm of the medial pterygoid blocks the opening action of the tensor veli palatini on the eustachian tube. Sore throat developing after exertion is a diagnostic aspect of CFS. Mild erythema is difficult to distinguish from variations of normal, and exudate is almost never encountered. Aphthous stomatitis is extremely common, as is periodontal disease. Both of these disorders are immunologically mediated. Patients often complain of coated tongues, which are only occasionally positive for candida. Taste disturbances, particularly hypogeusia, occur and are refractory to treatment.

Sometimes pain in the region of the anterior cervical lymph nodes may be caused by trigger points in the digastric muscle, which can be activated by bruxism and mouth breathing, as occurs in patients with nasal obstruction of various sorts. Digastric trigger points can be found in association with those in the medial pterygoid. They may be palpated by feeling behind the angle of the mandible upwards toward the earlobe, while pushing inward toward the neck muscle.

Lymphadenalgia, while more common than in the general population, is often confused with muscle tenderness and carotidynia. Some physicians are unfamiliar with the latter entity. The carotid bulb is enlarged and tender and palpation of the bulb intra-orally, on the floor of the mouth opposite the first molar, will elicit marked tenderness. Salivary gland disorders occur: primarily decreased production of saliva, but also various types of enlargement. Hypothyroidism, sometimes of the autoimmune variety, is often encountered, but goiter or thyroid masses are not. Lymphadenalgia could also be a result of alteration of neural input to the lymph nodes.[7]

The major abnormality related to the pulmonary system is chronic cough. This symptom may sometimes be related to asthma or chronic bronchitis, apparently more common in the CFS population, but also to postnasal drip or a hypersensitivity of the cough receptors. Dyspnea, either at rest or on exertion, is the most frequent complaint, but is probably mediated centrally. Asking the patient to hyperventilate in the office is helpful, although how to treat hyperventilation syndrome is problematic. Fifteen percent of CFS patients hyperventilate, which may cause bronchial constriction. Since the limbic system regulates the automatic control of respiration, hyperventilation could be a limbic dysregulation and may result in an overlap in the diagnosis of CFS and panic disorder. Hyperventilation is seen much more commonly in CFS patients with fibromyalgia.

Cardiac complaints primarily concern arrhythmias, usually supraventricular tachycardias. Although a large number of patients will have mitral valve prolapse, the role of this process in causing tachycardia in the CFS population is questionable. Some patients respond to beta blockers, but whether these treat a hyperadrenergic state rather than the myocardium or mitral valve is unclear. Primary myocardial disorders are uncommon in CFS although myocarditis does occur, usually viral. A limbic or paralimbic etiology for arrhythmias is much more attractive, particularly since these episodes may occur in the context of a panic disorder or what could be considered to be a forme fruste, e.g., "panic attack without anxiety." Chest pain does not usually seem to be pulmonary or cardiac, although coronary artery spasm and microvascular angina should be considered. CFS chest pain is more often esophageal or myofascial. Some patients will have symptoms of pleurodynia intermittently without fever or friction rub and with a normal chest X ray. "Costochondritis" per se does not occur, since there is no swelling of the costochondral junction. Another way to make the diagnosis of this disorder is by the "crowing rooster" maneuver to put the costochondral junctions on stretch. If this test is negative, one can assume that costochondral tenderness is secondary to tenderness of the sternalis muscle, the function of which is obscure. Chest pain can be produced by hyperventilation.

Gastrointestinal complaints are very common and symptoms of irritable bowel syndrome form an integral part of the CFS spectrum of symptoms. IBS should be included in the diagnostic criteria for a revised CFS case definition. We have discussed IBS previously. There are some helpful pointers on physical exam. The tenderness on abdominal palpation will sometimes resolve if the pressure of the examining fingers is continued. This sign does not occur with focal disease of the viscera. Myofascial etiologies for abdominal pain should always be looked for. Tenderness of the abdominal wall can be elicited by asking the patient to sit up halfway while palpation continues. Testing for trigger points in the external and internal obliques and in the iliocostalis will often be rewarding, as described by Travell and Simons.[8] Relief of the pain by local anesthetic infiltration may be helpful diagnostically, if one remembers that visceral disorders can cause somatic pain, and that the discomfort can sometimes be deceptively assuaged by trigger point elimination techniques. Patients with fibromyalgia are most prone to develop abdominal pain of muscular origin.

It is important to suspect pelvic disease. Perhaps the most common pelvic disorder in CFS is endometriosis, so common that I have postulated that the two disorders are related. Macrophages, the "vacuum cleaners" of the abdominal cavity, do not scavenge the normally refluxed endometrium which emits from Fallopian tube orifices during menstruation, and endometrial implants then occur. This defect in macrophage ingestion may occur in both CFS and endometriosis.

Adnexal masses and polycystic ovarian syndrome occur with greater frequency in CFS. Almost certainly these disorders are related to dysregulation of GnRH secretion, as has been discussed previously. Do not assume that adnexal masses are necessarily ovarian cysts in this population, however. Although the disorder is still uncommon, a much higher percentage of my patients in a CFS practice have developed ovarian carcinoma than I experienced while practicing family medicine. Some of these tumors have grown with startling rapidity. CFS patients continue to have CFS after their cancer treatment is completed.

Dysmenorrhea is also more common in CFS patients, even if endometriosis is not present. Although one could postulate that these women had excessive amounts of prostaglandins in their sloughed endometrium, a neural explanation is more plausible. A type of hollow visceral neuropathy could affect the uterus and/or there could be a disorder of descending pain modulation such as has been hypothesized to occur in fibromyalgia. Sometimes there will be diffuse tenderness on pelvic exam with no apparent cause.

A cause for pelvic pain which is often overlooked is pelvic floor tension myalgia. Patients with this disorder will often report dyspareunia and may be labeled as having a somatization disorder if they have a negative pelvic ultrasound and laparoscopy. If the pelvic floor, particularly the pyriformis muscle, is palpated in such a patient, it will be exquisitely tender and will respond well to trigger point injection or caudal epidural block. This type of pain sometimes begins after surgery in which the woman's legs are abducted for a time, such as a vaginal hysterectomy. It can be confused with lumbar radiculitis, since the sciatic nerve may be compressed between the sciatic notch and the pyriform muscle. Numerous other myofascial causes of pelvic, perineal, low back, and thigh pain are discussed in volume two of *The Trigger Point Manual* by Travell and Simons.[8] They are also common in CFS.

The primary genitourinary complaint in the male patient with CFS involves prostatic discomfort, frequency, and nocturia. Although many of these men are treated for prostatitis, very few of them have had a culture-proven infection, either of the urine or of prostatic fluid. Many have not had a three-glass test. My impression is that prostatitis, either chronic bacterial or abacterial, is considerably less common than prostatodynia. Acute bacterial prostatitis is seen no more frequently than in the general population. Prostatic tenderness is often detected in CFS patients, but induration or nodules with or without fever are not common. Alpha-blocking drugs such as prazosin (Minipress) or terazosin (Hytrin) are effective in diagnosis and treatment. Testalgia occurs infrequently, but is not accompanied by structural changes. This pain may be neuropathic. Intense scrotal and testicular pain was reported in a 9-year-old boy with a right parietal lobe seizure focus.[9] Lack of libido and erectile dysfunction are common complaints as well. When we have done nocturnal penile tumescence evaluation with Rigiscans, they have been abnormal.

The urethral syndrome in women is also more common in CFS. The causes of this disorder are numerous and include various kinds of inflammation, from chlamydia to interstitial cystitis. "Detrusor dyssynergia" is often found. It is treated with anticholinergic antispasmodics, alpha blockers (as in prostatodynia), and calcium channel blockers. A few patients will have intractable detrusor hyperflexia with incontinence. Such patients could be considered for intravesical capsaicin.[10] There may be tenderness of the muscles of the urogenital diaphragm, which would include the ischiocavernosus and the bulbocavernosus. These muscles are rarely examined, but could respond to the same sorts of trigger point elimination techniques as are used elsewhere.

Rectal exam is helpful in CFS to make the diagnosis of proctalgia fugax. This disorder is usually a myofascial pain syndrome of the levator ani. Many patients report sudden severe episodes of rectal pain which are usually brief, but may last as long as a half-hour or so. This problem, formerly consigned to the psychosomatic "wastebasket" until it was conceptualized and examined properly, is surprisingly common if one asks. It does not usually accompany burning rectal dysesthesias, another cardinal symptom of somatization disorder, although it may. Trigger point elimination techniques are helpful in treating proctalgia fugax. Levator ani trigger points, as well as those in the coccygeus muscle, can cause coccygeal pain, common in CFS. Stretch, post-isometric relaxation, massage, and high voltage pulsed galvanic stimulation are treatment modalities suitable for pelvic floor trigger points.

The number of musculoskeletal abnormalities related to fibromyalgia or myofascial pain syndrome is enormous. The physician must know how to elicit them on physical exam, or the patient may be diagnosed as having a somatoform pain disorder or a somatization disorder. The writings of Fishbain et al.[11] attest to the misdiagnosis of myofascial pain syndromes in the chronic pain patient because trigger point tenderness was not appropriately elicited by the examining physician. Other findings on musculoskeletal exam are not different than in the general population. Arthropathies are not common. EMGs are normal, not even suggesting focal muscle spasm or ongoing denervation. Sometimes bilateral leg pain may be due to a sensory neuropathy. Evidence for this hypothesis is that this symptom is often improved by capsaicin cream (Zostrix).

Neurologic exam is usually normal. Hard neurologic signs and muscle atrophy are rarely seen. Benign fasciculations are fairly common, as are tremors, usually of the essential variety, although iatrogenic hyperthyroidism is seen now and then. Parkinson's disease should be suspected in the middle-aged and older tremulous patient with central fatigue and cognitive dysfunction but no sore throat or flu symptoms. A Hallpike test is sometimes abnormal in vertiginous patients, as is the Romberg test. Muscle weakness is common, but is not accompanied by diffuse tenderness as would be seen in a myositis, and often it is not related to exertion as in the metabolic myopathies, but may get worse with repeated use as would be encountered in myasthenia gravis. Occasionally patients will have these disorders, and they should not be overlooked. Checking for temporal artery pulsations in selected CFS patients with headaches is a good idea, although cranial arteritis in this population is rare. Unsustained clonus is seen occasionally, as is deep tendon reflex asymmetry and anisocoria. I have two patients with persistently present extensor plantar reflexes and no other evidence of neurologic disease. Patients should be followed for the development of multiple sclerosis, or, more commonly in my experience, immune polyneuropathy. Diagnosis may be made more difficult by the rare patient with an elevated CPK for no apparent reason. Muscle biopsies in this group show evidence of mild denervation but are borderline normal. The Tensilon (edrophonium) test is sometimes positive in CFS and should not be interpreted as being diagnostic of myasthenia gravis. Muscle weakness in CFS may sometimes be treated with pyridostigmine bromide (Mestinon) when the usual diagnostic criteria for myasthenia gravis cannot be met. Surprisingly, Mestinon may alleviate mental "fogginess" as well, apparently by altering peripheral autonomic input to the CNS, or by inducing the adrenal glands to secrete more corticosteroids and catecholamines. It may also increase secretion of growth hormone.

Carpal tunnel syndrome (CTS) and thoracic outlet syndrome (TOS) are fairly common in CFS. The reason why the contents of the carpal tunnel should be compressed in CFS is obscure, as it is when CTS is associated with many other disorders. It is possible that the median nerve may have a heightened sensitivity to pressure. TOS is almost always related to muscle spasm and is seen in the setting of fibromyalgia. The usual maneuvers to elicit symptoms are applicable in CFS, although I have had few patients with symptoms severe enough to warrant ulnar nerve conduction velocities.

CFS patients often complain of easy bruisability or spontaneous ecchymoses. Clotting studies are usually normal, although some individuals have a mild thrombocytopenia which is apparently autoimmune. Platelet function studies are sometimes abnormal.

Psychiatric disorders are extremely common in a CFS population. Mood disorders, anxiety disorder, panic disorder, and borderline personality disorder are seen most frequently. I find somatization disorder to be rare, diagnosed without the previous caveats, as are related problems such as other somatoform disorders, hypochondriasis, and hysteria. It is important to obtain prior medical records. I have learned to suspect a psychiatric disorder in patients who claim to have no previous medical contact. An occasional delusional patient will believe that he has chronic fatigue syndrome caused by forces plotting against him, and a patient should be questioned about such false beliefs if his history sounds odd. Many patients could be diagnosed as having a post-traumatic stress disorder on the basis of a history of child abuse. Phobias are also common, especially agoraphobia and driving phobia.

DIAGNOSTIC TESTS

Although it is thought to be important to distinguish CFS from depression, as we have seen, this task is not too difficult unless one calls CFS an atypical depression, in which case it would have to be very atypical. The "Columbia criteria" are increasingly used to make the diagnosis of atypical depression. The patient must have (a) mood reactivity when depressed, (b) hyperphagia, hypersomnia, leaden paralysis of the limbs, or abnormal rejection sensitivity for most of his life (two of these for positive, one for probable).[12] These patients do not respond well to cyclic antidepressants, and do better with monoamine oxidase inhibitors, cognitive therapy,[13] and possibly selective serotonin reuptake inhibitors.[14] It could be a little harder to differentiate CFS from some cases of panic disorder, in which autonomic symptoms are more prominent. A case could be made that whether one makes the diagnosis of CFS or depression, panic disorder, or somatization depends on the physician's orientation, especially in patients who do not report flu-like symptoms, sore throat, worsening of symptoms the next day by exercise, and alcohol intolerance. The physician evaluating CFS patients should have a good understanding of anxiety. A useful primer is *Panic Disorder in the Medical Setting,* by Wayne Katon, published in 1989 by the U.S. Department of Health and Human Services. These diagnostic issues are not just hair-splitting since treatment decisions must be made and health and disability insurance issues depend on whether the patient has a "nervous or mental disorder." It is thus often necessary to do diagnostic tests beyond what has been recommended by the NIH, even though they may be labeled "experimental." Furthermore, since CFS appears to be multi-causal, it would be of value to know which patients had a virus detected.

Identification of viruses should be very helpful, since nervous and mental disorders are not usually considered to be associated with infections, although there is increasing evidence that some cases of schizophrenia are. At the present time the most available tests are cultures for the CFS-associated retroviruses, and polymerase chain reactions for EBV, CMV, and HHV-6. Although PCR is quite helpful, its reliability is determined by the sensitivity of the assay, which can be modulated by the pathologist. False positives occur, and one wonders whether herpes viruses should be treated with antiviral agents on the basis of a polymerase chain reaction result without physical signs of infection, especially when potentially toxic agents such as ganciclovir or foscarnet might be used. Ribavirin has also been used by some. Such tests have little role in clinical decision making at present, although investigation of potential viral candidates continues.

A positive culture is better diagnostic information, especially when the virus being cultured is not seen in apparently normal people, as CMV can be. HHV-6 can be detected by monoclonal antibodies in an experimental giant cell assay, although once again, there are ambiguities about whether this virus should be treated. Are the potential benefits greater than the risks? Can the morbidity of CFS be improved by decreasing the load of transactivating co-viruses (as in AIDS)? Should a lumbar puncture be done if blood results are negative? These questions are currently unanswered. Rubella viremia could be investigated if symptoms began subsequent to rubella vaccination. Other forms of post-vaccinial CFS seem to be immunologically, not virally, mediated.

Detecting viral gene products, such as glycoproteins, is another method of viral diagnosis. No such products have yet been identified in CFS. An assay for the gp120 antigen has been developed. Antibodies to gp120 are negative in CFS.

Viral antibody titers are virtually useless in CFS. There appears to be an impairment of the suppression of antibody production, particularly to herpes viruses, in CFS. At present, I do not order these tests.

I do order titers for Lyme disease and (sometimes) toxoplasmosis. I will treat the patient with IgG and IgM antibody to *borrelia burgdorferi* on repeat testing even when there is no history of the typical rash and no findings of arthritis. The morbidity of the patients I see is so great, and the risk of oral or IV antibiotics so small, that a therapeutic trial is often justified. Sometimes it works, other times not. The issue is further confused by the fact that patients with unequivocal Lyme disease can still have a CFS picture after treatment which has cured their arthritis. The common neurologic abnormalities in Lyme disease, radiculitis, meningitis, and cranial neuritis are not frequently seen in a CFS patient. I see an occasional patient with persistently elevated IgM and IgG antibodies to toxoplasmosis. Thus far I have not treated these patients and have not seen any progression to the physical signs caused by the organism. I have referred some of these patients to infectious disease specialists, but they are perplexed also.

Isolation of intestinal parasites by stool exam and antibody titers is often valuable. Some cases of apparent CFS have been cured by anti-parasitic therapy, as has been described by Leo Galland.[15] I have not used purged stools or special laboratories, but do order anti-giardia antibodies and detection of giardia antigen in stool. I have done numerous rectal mucus swabs and have abandoned the procedure because of its low yield. The mechanism by which intestinal parasites can cause CFS is unknown, but may be cytokine-mediated. Sometimes a patient will have "non-pathogenic" parasites isolated. Current dogma is that these organisms should not be treated if they do not cause gastrointestinal symptoms, but if they cause an immune response which could produce CFS, then perhaps they should be treated.

A New Zealand researcher reports abnormalities in red cell morphology in CFS that could be associated with a low sed rate.[16] Although these findings have been called artifactual by some, one of the defects ("cup forms") often responds to vitamin B_{12} injections, which also are reported to relieve symptoms. This morphologic abnormality suggests a membrane defect which may be resolved by a methyl group donor. Trials of the methyl donor S-adenosylmethionine in FM have been beneficial.[17]

Routine lab tests include CBC, urinalysis, chemical profile, antinuclear antibody, rheumatoid factor, thyroid stimulating hormone, HIV serology, and serum ferritin. CFS and panic disorder patients often have significant elevations in serum cholesterol from premorbid levels.[18] Possible mechanisms of hypercholesterolemia in CFS include production of IgM or IgG that binds to heparin, thereby decreasing activity of lipoprotein lipase. Heparin is an attractive therapy in CFS if mast cell abnormalities are suspected, but heparin has been fairly unsuccessful in the treatment of interstitial cystitis, thought by some to be related to bladder mast cell dysfunction. Hypercholesterolemia in CFS could also be caused by increased secretion and decreased catabolism of very low density lipoproteins, perhaps due to altered function of BAT. IL-1, acting either peripherally or centrally, has produced elevations of free fatty acids in mice, without acting directly on the pancreas.[19] CFS patients do not have increased atherosclerosis, however.

I will not discuss various tests of immune activation in great detail. The sed rate is often very low. Immune complexes and positive anti-nuclear antibodies are encountered very frequently. Anti-lymphocyte antibodies are negative. Elevated levels of various cytokines and their receptors are often seen. Some researchers maintain that these have prognostic significance and can also serve as a measure of disease activity, but I am not so sure, at least in my patient population. The multitest CMI (cell-mediated immunity) for delayed-type hypersensitivity can be useful, especially when the patient is initially anergic. I am not sure how to use information such as low (or high) natural killer cell function or levels of the soluble CD8 receptor. I do not find the mitogen stimulation test or T & B cell subset analysis to be helpful. Paul Cheney has a number of CFS patients with low CD4 counts that he is following. For the most part, they do not differ clinically from other CFS patients, although two have opportunistic infections. The etiology of the CD4 depression is unclear, but is thought to be related to a CFS-associated viral agent, perhaps in combination with one or more transactivating viruses or other microbes. The role of limbic regulation of immune function in these patients is uncertain. It is possible that the low CD4 counts reported in some CFS patients may not necessarily be due to viral infection of this lymphocyte to population, but may be related to altered limbic regulation of the innervation of lymphoid organs, so that CD4 cells may not develop properly.[20,21] Cytokines, thymic hormones, and extra-thymic influences via the limbic system and pituitary regulate the secretory function of thymic epithelial cells and the stepwise evolution of T-cells and induction of T-cell receptors.[22,23] Limbic modulation of nerves innervating the thymus is possible.[24] I have not ordered tests for cytokine generation by lymphocytes. I am concerned that there may be wide variability between labs in reporting results of many of these more esoteric tests of immune function.

A broad spectrum of diseases–infectious, autoimmune, nutritional, congenital, and lymphoproliferative–may be associated with a fall in CD4 cell count. Drugs (e.g., corticosteroids), old age and pregnancy can also cause low CD4 counts. Sometimes CD4 counts can fall because of sequestration of these cells in the reticuloendothelial system as a result of infection.[25] Lymphopenia of a T-cell subset could also be produced by a virally encoded superantigen,[26] or decreased production of a specific growth factor.[27]

The main serum cytokine elevations noted in the literature have been IL-1 alpha, IL-2, alpha interferon, and IL-6. A recent report, which noted elevations in serum transforming growth factor-beta (TGF-beta) also included release of cytokines in peripheral blood mononuclear cell cultures.[28] Elevations in IL-1 alpha were reported in 35% of the Ampligen patients, and correlated with a good response to treatment. I attempted to measure most of these cytokines several years ago with James Peter, Michael Palladino, and John Martin, but found the results too inconsistent to be of clinical utility. Since serum inhibitors of cytokines are common, the measurement of mRNA for such transmitters will be more valuable. My initial hypothesis was that CFS is a cytokine-mediated illness, but cytokine measurement in CFS and FM, as of now, is not useful. In sub-typing CFS, mRNA techniques may help. I published an hypothesis of CFS as a TGF-beta excess syndrome several years ago.[29] The effect of cytokines in the brain can be profound at very low levels and can cause suppression or activation of peripheral immune responses. Immune suppression has been described with IL-1 infused in picogram quantities into the lateral ventricle of rats.[30] These effects were blocked by infusion of alpha-melanocyte stimulating hormone (alpha-MSH), a known IL-1 antagonist. Infusion of IL-1 at these levels did not elevate body temperature and may have actually decreased it. Plasma corticosteroid levels were elevated in the infused animals (unlike CFS patients), but 50% of the immune suppression noted in intact animals was seen in adrenalectomized animals, probably mediated by the sympathetic nervous system. Cellular immune responses in splenic lymphocytes were suppressed by a lower dose of IL-1 than that needed to suppress the function of peripheral lymphocytes. Modulation of an autonomic neural pathway from brain to spleen, as demonstrated by Felten et al.,[31] was suggested.

The roles of IL-1 alpha and beta in the brain have recently been reviewed by N. J. Rothwell.[32] These subtypes of IL-1 have similar effects for the most part, but may exert them by different mechanisms, and produce them at much lower concentrations than in the periphery. Central actions of IL-1 as listed include the following:

1. Local effects in brain: altered EEG and neuronal activity, inhibition of long-term potentiation, cortical inhibitory postsynaptic function, neurotransmitter release/turnover, induction of nerve growth factor (NGF), self-induction (of IL-1 beta), astrogliosis, and neovascularization. IL-1 further opens the chloride channel of the $GABA_A$ receptor when the receptor is already occupied

by GABA.[33] IL-1 is probably involved in antagonizing vasospasm by stimulating nitric oxide synthase.

2. Metabolic actions: fever, increased metabolic rate (thermogenesis), sympathetic activation of brown fat, hypophagia, and altered gastric function.

3. Endocrine actions: hypothalamic-pituitary hormone release (CRH, GnRH, TSH, ACTH), pituitary-adrenal activation, and insulin release.

4. Behavioral actions: sleep, and sickness behavior (e.g., reduced exploration). Central IL-1 may also decrease pain.[34]

5. Immune actions: peripheral IL-6 release, decreased peripheral IL-2 production, reduced natural killer cell activity, leukocytosis, and hepatic acute phase protein synthesis.

Some of these actions appear to apply to CFS and others not. The idea that CNS cytokines are involved in the pathogenesis of CFS is very persuasive, however, and since so many transmitter substances may be involved in the modulation of IL-1 activity, the role of this cytokine cannot be dismissed. As in peripheral blood, CNS cytokine measurement has yielded conflicting results. Concentrations of CSF IL-1 inhibitory substances have not been reported.

Laboratories are looking for abnormalities in lymphocyte metabolism. Perhaps the most useful assay will be for $2',5'$ oligo-adenylate synthetase/RNase L, which was significantly elevated in Ampligen responders. This test is not generally available. A protein kinase C deficit has been noted in the failure of lymphocytes from patients with fibromyalgia to generate IL-2.[35] The p15E retroviral envelope protein impairs IL-1 signal transduction by blocking protein kinase C.[36] This finding is of interest since tung oil, a phorbol ester (which stimulates protein kinase C) has been implicated in the etiology of CFS in some patients. Serine proteases can be demonstrated by immunogold staining in natural killer cells stimulated with IL-2 and are thought to be the means by which those cells destroy targets. NK cells from CFS patients with low NK function are being investigated to see if these enzymes are deficient.[37] I generally measure quantitative immunoglobulins to check for monoclonal gammopathies as well as deficiencies, particularly of IgA, since IgA deficient patients are at risk for receiving gamma globulin exogenously. I have stopped measuring anti-IgA antibodies because they are too expensive, and I find IgG subclass levels and response to pneumococcal vaccine to be an academic exercise which has little bearing on patient response. Abnormal results in these tests may, however, convince insurance companies to pay for gamma globulin therapy on the basis of an immunodeficiency. I sometimes do studies to assess the integrity of the hypothalamic-pituitary-adrenal (HPA) axis. Dexamethasone-suppression tests are usually normal. ACTH stimulation tests are sometimes abnormal but treatment of the patient with corticosteroids based on this result is only occasionally helpful. CRH is not generally available, but ACTH reserve could be tested indirectly by a metyrapone test. The few thyrotropin releasing hormone (TRH) tests I have done have usually shown a blunted TSH response. Patients with primary fibromyalgia syndrome responded to 400 micrograms of TRH with a lower than normal secretion of TSH and thyroid hormone, as well as a significantly higher increase in prolactin.[38] Baseline prolactins are occasionally elevated, but not enough to order them routinely. Patients sometimes have galactorrhea with or without hyperprolactinemia, and none of my patients has had a pituitary adenoma. Neuroendocrine dysfunction in CFS is discussed in the next chapter, but is best assessed with the patient in a stressed, not a resting, state since CFS may, in one sense, be viewed as a dysregulation of homeostatic mechanisms.

BRAIN FUNCTION TESTS

I believe that tests of brain function are quite helpful. The best one may be the SPECT (single photon emission computerized tomography) scan. In this procedure we administer Xenon 133 by inhalation and do a computerized scan of cerebral blood flow using a brain-dedicated SPECT scanner. Using other types of SPECT scanners does not provide adequate resolution. We then ask the patient to perform cardiopulmonary exercise testing, looking for a lowered anaerobic threshold, respiratory alkalosis suggesting hyperventilation, and irregular respiratory rhythms at maximum exercise suggesting disordered central regulation of respiration. Exercise-induced electrocardiographic signs of ischemia in this fairly young population suggest dysregulation of vasomotor tone, or "vasoregulatory asthenia." After physiologic parameters return to baseline we repeat the Xenon 133 study and may also do one with technetium 99m-hexamethylpropylene-amine oxime (HMPAO). Pre- and post-exercise neuroendocrine measurements are performed and if the patient is able to return in the next day or two, we omit the technetium study and do another Xenon 133 scan. Although we have not completed testing all comparison groups, SPECT results are quite distinctive. There is resting hypoperfusion in the anterior temporal lobes, more often seen in the right. There is also hypoperfusion in the prefrontal cortex. The hypoperfusion is usually worsened by exercise, the opposite of what is seen in normal subjects.

We have recently compared groups of depressed and non-depressed CFS patients over the age of 45 to a comparison group of patients with major depressive disorder. The technetium HMPAO SPECT scans of the depressed patients showed bilateral orbitofrontal hypoperfusion, left greater than right. The CFS patients had only right dorsolateral prefrontal hypoperfusion rather than orbitofrontal. These results were highly significant. CFS patients who met DSM-III-R criteria for major depressive disorder did not differ from those who did not. CFS patients with FM had significantly greater regional cerebral hypoperfusion than those who did not have FM. The implications of this study are perhaps that amygdalar lesions are more involved in depression while hippocampal lesions are pathogenetic in CFS, and that hemispheric asymmetry is present in CFS. To quote Joaquin Fuster:

> Nauta (1964) pointed out, on the basis of primate data, that the orbitofrontal cortex is connected mainly to the amygdala complex and related subcortical structures, whereas the dorsal prefrontal convexity is connected to the hippocampal and parahippocampal cortex . . . The functional significance of prefrontal connections with the limbic system is still unclear, but in all probability these connections involve the prefrontal cortex in neural functions that maintain and protect the organism's internal milieu. The reciprocal connection between the dorsolateral prefrontal cortex and the hippocampus, through

the entorhinal cortex, are probably involved in cognitive functions . . . [39]

If the abnormalities seen on SPECT are primarily related to the regulation of regional cerebral blood flow, a differential expression of the potentially vasoconstrictive IL-1ra mRNA[40] may be involved. Other IL-1 inhibitors, such as TGF-beta and IL-10, which also inhibit the vasodilator nitric oxide, should be considered as well (see Conclusion).

A PET scan study of patients with major depressive disorder showed reduced metabolic activity in the left anterior cingulate and the left dorsolateral prefrontal cortex. Increased blood flow in the cerebellar vermis was also noted.[41] A SPECT scan using ^{99m}Tc-HMPAO in major depression showed reduced uptake in the temporal, inferior frontal, and parietal areas of the neocortex and in the basal ganglia and thalamus. Those who were psychotically depressed had relatively greater uptake in the cingulate and dorsolateral frontal cortex, when compared to other patients with major depression.[42] There have been brain SPECT studies using ^{99m}Tc-HMPAO in CFS. Regional cerebral blood flow was decreased in 65% of patients in the frontal regions, in 35% in the temporal regions, in 53% in the parietal regions, and in 38% in the occiptal regions in one of these experiments.[43] Forty percent of the patients also had reduced cerebral blood flow in the basal ganglia. This group did not find lateralization of hypoperfusion, and found reduced regional cerebral blood flow in certain areas (basal ganglia, occipital cortex) where we virtually never see it. The resolution of the SPECT scans in this experiment was not as good as ours and (a) the CFS patients were not stratified due to age, and lateralization may be confined to those over 45, and (b) technical factors involving attenuation of the signal from the basal ganglia, since they are deeper than the cortex, make interpretation of basal ganglia blood flow by SPECT very difficult. We sometimes see posterior parietal hypoperfusion in CFS brain SPECT scans, and it may be that the determination of the boundaries of the occipital cortex in this study were wider than we use.

One of the minor criteria in the CDC case definition for CFS is severe post-exercise fatigue lasting 24 hours or longer. This symptom is reflected in post-exercise SPECT scans which usually have much greater degrees of hypoperfusion than baseline, as seen in Xenon 133 scans done the same day and the next. Limited numbers of post-treatment scans suggest that improvement in regional cerebral hypoperfusion is correlated with lessening of symptoms. It appears that the hypoperfusion is a reflection of an underlying metabolic abnormality, since agents that increase cerebral blood flow do not reliably improve CFS symptoms. The temporal lobes and orbitofrontal cortex are part of the limbic system. The dorsolateral prefrontal cortex is a heteromodal association area related to the paralimbic cortex. Brain SPECT allows a quantification of functional abnormality which is not based solely on self-report. It has significant relevance to the work of Renoux on lateralization of cortical immune function[44] as well as to lateralization of $5HT_2$ receptors.[45]

Topographic brain mapping with evoked responses is almost always abnormal in CFS patients. The temporal lobes, left more than right, are most frequently abnormal on visual and auditory evoked response measurement by BEAM (brain electrical activity mapping), which compares these results in 36 millisecond segments to a normal population and then calculates the difference from this group, which to be significant is two or more standard deviations from normal. The technology of the BEAM scanner allows evoked response data to be examined in 2 millisecond segments if desired. Paper EEG, computerized EEG, and somatosensory evoked responses are usually normal. There is often an absent or asymmetric n-120 wave in the VER, thought to indicate attentional disorders, and a similarly abnormal p-180 wave in the VER, suggesting an encephalopathic process. BEAM abnormalities are seen more frequently in other cortical areas than on SPECT.

Evoked response testing in the usual manner (without BEAM), can also be abnormal. The types of abnormalities may help in distinguishing CFS from multiple sclerosis, which in its early stages may be quite similar to CFS. We have found a highly significant abnormality in the P100 wave in the auditory evoked responses of 12 out of 12 CFS patients, suggesting a hippocampal localization. A group from London has reported abnormalities in latency or amplitude of the P300 wave in the cognitive event-related potentials but not in sensory-related potentials of about 50% of 37 CFS patients tested.[46] MS patients have more widespread derangements in evoked responses and should be able to be distinguished from individuals with CFS on this basis as well as several others.

PET (positron emission tomography) scans are also abnormal in a distinctive fashion, implicating limbic structures most frequently as being hypometabolic. The medial frontal lobe, the hippocampus, amygdala, and cingulate gyrus are usually involved as are the anterior caudate nucleus, superior colliculus, and areas of the parietal lobe. Sometimes the premotor cortex and anterior cerebellum are also hypometabolic. PET scans utilize radioactive fluorodeoxyglucose which is injected intravenously prior to computerized scanning. The expense of the test and duration of action of the tracer preclude doing the type of exercise testing that we do with SPECT scans. The limits of resolution of the PET scanner that I use are 6 mm, not good enough to image small structures such as the nucleus accumbens. Newer PET scanners will be able to resolve down to 2 mm, a distinct improvement. Both PET and SPECT technology will be revolutionized by the use of isotopes which label receptors. The multiple serotonin and dopamine receptors are of interest, and compounds to label them are available now. We shall start using them shortly.

Magnetic resonance imaging of the brain demonstrates increased numbers of frontoparietal subcortical high signal intensity lesions in young people that are not necessarily in the characteristic locations for demyelinating disease. These UBOs (unidentified bright objects) are of uncertain etiology, and the neuroradiologist must be sensitized to their detection. They are often ignored as a normal variant of no significance. UBOs were an indicator of a positive response to Ampligen. Hippocampal volumes may be reduced, implying a poorer prognosis, and special coronal cuts must be ordered to assess this cortical area. A technique recently described is measurement of cerebral blood flow by MRI. How MRI blood flow measurement would compare with SPECT and whether post-exercise MRI blood flow studies would be feasible remains to be seen. A group of CFS patients are being examined with a new technique, magnetoencephalography. We are studying brain metabolism with magnetic resonance spectroscopy, a tool with great potential for studying tissue composition in disorders of function such as CFS.[47] Preliminary results indicate adequate glutamate/glutamine levels in the occipital cortex, a region which is normal on CFS SPECT and PET scans. Glutamate/glutamine levels are reduced in the frontoparietal region. This finding could relate to decreased activity of nitric oxide synthase, which catalyzes the production of nitric oxide from L-arginine. However, low levels of glutamate/glutamine would suggest an impairment of glutamate storage, since MRS findings do not reflect kinetics or secretion. This result is being investigated further. Nitric oxide functions as a retrograde neurotransmitter, diffusing from a post-synaptic neuron with glutamate receptors into the interstitium. Nitric oxide then diffuses only into pre-synaptic neurons that are firing and augments their secretion of glutamate. This mechanism of glutamatergic secretory augmentation has been described in long-term potentiation, but may occur in other situations (see Conclusion).

Neuropsychological testing is important diagnostically as well as in measuring functional impairment to determine the degree of disability. Medical insurance sometimes will not cover such testing even if it is quite abnormal and diagnostic of an organic dementia. In our patients it reliably differentiates depression as well as other dementing disorders from CFS. Since neuropsychologists vary in their training and approach, computerized testing methods, such as we use, are being developed so that the quality and process can be standardized as well as reduced in cost. Superficial kinds of cognitive testing, such as the Mini-Mental Status exam, are usually normal. As has been discussed previously, CFS patients are prone to overestimating their cognitive abilities. Their making of new memories is extremely fragile and disrupted by proactive interference. They do not benefit from memory cues. The making of new memories is easily disturbed by increasing the amount of information presented. Depressed patients underestimate their cognitive abilities and have normal testing, although their response time is slowed. On the basis of test results indicating a hippocampal lesion, we may diagnose our patients as having temporolimbic dysfunction, amnestic disorder, or metabolic encephalopathy.

Other types of psychological testing instruments are also used, and the literature is proliferating rapidly. It may be helpful to know if there was a premorbid psychiatric disorder, and if so, what kind. The Diagnostic Interview Schedule (DIS) has been adapted for use in medical patients. It is mainly a research tool. It is a highly structured "no brainer" algorithm which asks specific questions about each symptom endorsed. Psychiatric symptoms and onset of fatigue can be dated. There are problems using the DIS in CFS because the need to modify it to rate a medical illness with cognitive dysfunction may decrease its validity.

We use the Minnesota Multiphasic Personality Inventory (MMPI-2). It is the best validated of all psychologic tests. We have found there is a unique and probably diagnostic profile in CFS: elevations in scales 1, 2, 3, 4, 7, and 8.[48] Unless the interpreting psychologist is familiar with this pattern, the test results may be misinterpreted. This pattern suggests chronic illness and cognitive dysfunction.

It is of value to screen CFS patients for psychiatric problems using standardized instruments, both for clinical information and for stratification in a research or epidemiologic paradigm. Test results must be interpreted with caution, however, since mood disorders may be overdiagnosed in a population with chronic illness and neuropsychologic impairment. Our patients receive:

1. *Symptom Checklist 90:* a 90-item, 5-point self-rating scale. It has nine dimensional scales: somatization, obsessive-compulsive, interpersonal sensitivity, depression, anxiety, hostility, phobic anxiety, paranoid ideation, and psychoticism.
2. *Beck Depression Inventory:* a 63-item, 4-point self-rating scale indicative of a person's feelings in the past week, including the day of administration.
3. *Beck Anxiety Inventory:* a 21-item, 4-point adjective self-rating scale that indicates the severity of the anxiety felt during the past week, including the day of administration.
4. *Karnofsky Performance Scale:* a self-rating scale from 0 to 100 indicating the ability of the patient to perform activities of daily living.
5. *Somatosensory Amplification Scale:* a 10-item self-rating scale which notes the presence of symptoms associated with somatization.
6. *Columbia Criteria for Atypical Depression:* assessed by the physician.

These tests provide much useful information at little cost, and can be scored rapidly and interpreted by the physician. The findings can be integrated with other clinical data and may indicate the need for further investigation.

Are CFS patients with premorbid psychiatric diagnoses more chronic in their course and more resistant to treatment? Experience might suggest that this is so, but the results of the Ampligen experiment do not support this impression. Most studies suggest, however, that premorbid psychiatric illness is more common in CFS patients than in comparison groups with other medical diagnoses, such as rheumatoid arthritis or neuromuscular disorders. It has been suggested that this CFS group may be more prone to "somatize" psychological distress and are thus subject to the "biologic" effects of depression.[49] This tendency to report high levels of somatic symptoms has been called "somatosensory amplification." Some view this as a perceptual style amenable to change through cognitive and behavioral interventions. Using this paradigm, those with no premorbid psychiatric illness and an acute onset of CFS symptoms may have a cytokine-mediated illness. The unifying concept of a limbic encephalopathy appears to be a new one, and could explain somatosensory amplification as a dysfunction of the insula or other paralimbic areas, as previously discussed. Rats with a central defect in the secretion of CRH demonstrate behavior compatible with somatosensory amplification as well as a failure of immune suppression in response to inflammatory stimuli. These rats provide a model of the relationship between stress and the immune system.[50]

Another method to evaluate the CFS patient which has not received attention in the literature is the functional capacity evaluation. Functional capacity evaluation (FCE) is "an assessment of functional ability to perform work activities which include the physical demand factors on which the Dictionary of Occupational Titles is based."

The functional capacity evaluation done on my patients is an intensive 5- to 7-hour assessment. The evaluation involves standardized physical and cognitive testing including the following:

- Static strength testing utilizing NIOSH strength standards
- Dynamic strength testing utilizing Stover Snook norms

- Review of critical job demands
- Range of motion evaluations
- Manual strength evaluations
- Test of symptom magnification
- Dictionary of Occupational Title physical demand levels
- Cardiopulmonary assessment–3-minute step test
- O'Connor finger dexterity test
- Minnesota manual dexterity evaluation
- Activities of daily living assessment
- Computerized functional capacity checklist
- Neurobehavioral cognitive status examination (NCSE)
- Employee aptitude survey (EAS)
- Raven standard progressive matrices
- Symbol digit modalities test
- Valpar work component work samples

An assessment and recommendations follow the evaluation. The report analyzes the patient's ability to perform the critical job demands required by his/her job description. It is, in essence, a comparison of the patient's present physical and cognitive status to the physical and cognitive demands of his/her work and activities of daily living, including self care. The FCE is given to patients with CFS and is a major determinant in setting up an individualized work-hardening program or assessing the patient's ability to return to work and to perform self-care. The patient is physically present at the testing location for 5 to 7 hours. Breaks are allowed as needed. His ability to participate in the lengthy evaluation is observed and considered when recommendations are made. By ordering this evaluation I am provided with a definitive baseline of the patient's functional ability. This information is objective and invaluable for determining a patient's present and future work capacity and for determination of the level of disability. The evaluation includes an extensive 15- to 20-page report with specific findings from standardized tests, the assignment of a Dictionary of Occupational Title physical demand level, and a summary of the patient's ability and potential ability.

Common findings of an FCE in CFS are significant deterioration in dynamic, repetitive strength testing, marked memory impairment with relative preservation of other cognitive functions on the NCSE, and performance capabilities in the lower (or lowest) percentiles when compared with occupational norms. Most patients relapse for several days after the evaluation. We have not tested anyone whom we thought was malingering.

OVERVIEW

I know of no other mechanism than a limbic encephalopathy by which the common diagnostic constellation of CFS, FM, IBS, panic disorder, dysthymia, night sweats, depression, hippocampal cognitive disorder, nasal allergy, sleep disorder, sore throats, tinnitus, vertigo, intermittent blurred vision, PMS, alopecia, and endometriosis (to name a few) could be produced. Variations in the manner in which the limbic system is dysfunctional could account for symptom predominance. Viruses can alter the function of neurons or neuronal networks in a manner similar to developmental abnormalities and environmental stressors. Secondary adrenal insufficiency due to a central mechanism relating to CRH deficiency could also be responsible for many CFS symptoms and will be discussed in the next chapter. There are some patients whose disorder may be a genetic, acquired, or learned somatosensory amplification. These categories may, of course, overlap. I am currently exploring the idea that interference with central IL-1 beta action is characteristic of CFS. It may become apparent that, just as the limbic system integrates function on a neuroanatomic basis, so does a balance of cytokines does so from a neurochemical perspective.

REFERENCES

1. Manu P, Lane TJ, Mathews DA. Somatization disorder in patients with chronic fatigue. *Psychosomatics* 30(4): 388-394, 1989.

2. Schluederberg A, Straus SE, Peterson P, Blumenthal S, Komaroff AL, Spring SB, Landay A, Buchwald D. NIH Conference. Chronic fatigue syndrome research. Definition and medical outcome assessment. *Ann Int Med* 117(4): 325-331, 1992.

3. Landay AL, Jessop C, Lennette ET, Levy JA. Chronic fatigue syndrome: clinical condition associated with immune activation. *Lancet* 338: 707-712, 1991.

4. Carter WA. Presented at: 3rd Interscience Conference on Antimicrobial Agents and Chemotherapy. Chicago, October 1, 1991.

5. Sharpe MC, et al. Report of a consensus meeting, Oxford, 23 March 1990. A report–chronic fatigue syndrome: guidelines for research. *J R Soc Med* 24: 118-119, 1991.

6. Chessick RD, Bolin RR. Psychiatric study of patients with psychomotor seizures. *J Nerv Ment Dis* 134: 72-79, 1962.

7. Bellinger DL, Lorton D, Felten SY, Felten DL. Innervation of lymphoid organs and implications in development, aging, and autoimmunity. *Int J Immunopharmacol* 14(3): 329-344, 1992.

8. Travell J, Simons D. *Myofascial Pain and Dysfunction: The Trigger Point Manual.* New York, Williams and Wilkins, 1983.

9. Mesulam M-M. *Principles of Behavioral Neurology.* Philadelphia, FA Davis, 1985.

10. Fowler CJ, Jewkes D, McDonald WI, Lynn B, de Groat WC. Intravesical capsaicin for neurogenic bladder dysfunction. *Lancet* 339: 1239, 1992.

11. Fishbain DA, Goldberg M, Rosomoff RS, Rosomoff H. Chronic pain patients and the non-organic physical sign of nondermatomal sensory abnormalities (NDSA). *Psychosomatics* 32(3): 294-302, 1991.

12. Liebowitz MR, Quitkin FM, Steward JW, McGrath PH, Harrison WM, Markowitz JS, Rabkin JG, Tricamo E, Goetz DM, Klein DF. Antidepressant specificity in atypical depression. *Arch Gen Psychiatry* 45: 129-138, 1988.

13. Mercier MA, Stewart JW, Quitkin FM. A pilot sequential study of cognitive therapy and pharmacotherapy of atypical depression. *J Clin Psychiatry* 53(5): 166-170, 1992.

14. Stewart JW, Quitkin FM, Klein DF. The pharmacotherapy of minor depression. *Am J Psychiatry* 46(1): 23-36, 1992.

15. Galland L. The effect of systemic microbes on systemic immunity. In: Jenkins R and Mowbray JF (eds.). *Postviral Fatigue Syndromes.* Chichester, John Wiley, 1991.

16. Newbold HL. Vitamin B-12: placebo or neglected therapeutic tool? *Med Hypotheses* 28: 155-164, 1989.

17. Jacobsen S, Danneskjold-Samsoe B, Andersen RB. Oral S-adenosylmethionine in primary fibromyalgia. Double-blind clinical evaluation. *Scand J Rheumatol* 20: 294-302, 1991.

18. Bajwa WK, Asnis GM, Sanderson WC, Irfan A, Van Praag NM. High cholesterol levels in patients with panic disorder. *Am J Psychiatry* 149: 376-378, 1992.

19. Besedovsky HO, del Rey A. Immune-neuroendocrine circuits: integrative role of cytokines. *Frontiers Neuroendocrinol* 15(1): 61-94, 1992.

20. Meluche S, Lamorre D, Zerbib A, Fleury SG, Sekaly R-P. CD4. In: *Encyclopedia of Immunology.* Roitt IM, Delves PJ (eds.), London, Academic Press, 1992.

21. Bellinger DL, Lorton D, Felten SY, Felten DL. Innervation of lymphoid organs and implications in development, aging, and autoimmunity. *Int J Immunopharmacol* 14(3): 329-344, 1992.

22. Hadden JH. Thymic endocrinology. *Int J Immunopharmacol* 14(3): 345-352, 1992.

23. Hadden JH, Hadden EM, Coffey RG. First and second messengers in the development and function of thymus-dependent lymphocytes. In: *Psychoneuroimmunology,* second edition. Ader R, Felten DF, Cohen N (eds.), San Diego: Academic Press, 1990.

24. Felten SY, Felten DL. Innervation of lymphoid tissue. In: *Psychoneuroimmunology,* second edition. Ader R, Felten DF, Cohen N (eds.), San Diego: Academic Press, 1990.

25. Soriano V, Hewlett I, Heredia A, Pedreira J, Gutierrez M, Bravo R, Castro A, Gonzalez-Lahoz J. Idiopathic CD4+ T-lymphopenia. *Lancet* 340: 607-608, 1992.

26. Drake CG, Kotzin BL. Superantigens: biology, immunology, and potential role in disease. *J Clin Immunol* 12(3): 149-161, 1992.

27. Brenneman D. Neuroimmune interactions: implications for neuro-AIDS and neurodevelopment. Presented at: The Seminar in Behavioral Neuroimmunology, Los Angeles, UCLA School of Medicine, November 2, 1992.

28. Chao CC, Janoff EN, Hu S, Thomas K, Gallagher M, Tsong M, Peterson PK. Altered cytokine release in peripheral blood mononuclear cell cultures from patients with the chronic fatigue syndrome. *Cytokine* 3(4): 292-298, 1991.

29. Goldstein, JA. *Chronic Fatigue Syndrome: The Struggle for Health.* Los Angeles: Chronic Fatigue Syndrome Institute, 1990.

30. Weiss JM, Sundar SK, Becker KJ, Cierpial MA. Behavioral and neural influences on cellular immune responses: effects of stress and interleukin-1. *J Clin Psychiatry* 50(5) (suppl): 43-52,1989.

31. Felten SY, Felten DL. Innervation of lymphoid tissue. In: Ader R, Felten DF, Cohen N (eds). *Psychoneuroimmunology,* second edition. San Diego, Academic Press, 1991.

32. Rothwell NJ. Functions and mechanisms of interleukin-1 in the brain. *Trends Pharmacol Sci* 12(11): 430-436, 1991.

33. Dinarello CA. Interleukin-1 and interleukin-1 antagonism. *Blood* 77(8): 1627-1652, 1991.

34. Oppenheim JJ, Shevach EM. Immunophysiology: The role of cells and cytokines in immunity and inflammation. New York, Oxford University Press, 1990.

35. Hader N, Rimon D, Kinarty A, Lahat N. Altered interleukin-2 secretion in patients with primary fibromyalgia syndrome. *Arth Rheum* 34(7): 866-871, 1991.

36. Dinarello CA. Interleukin-1 and interleukin-1 antagonism. *Blood* 77(8): 1627-1652, 1991.

37. Vojdani A. Personal communication, 1992.

38. Neeck G, Riedel W. Thyroid function in patients with fibromyalgia syndrome. *J Rheumatol* 19: 1120-1122, 1992.

39. Fuster JM. *The prefrontal cortex: anatomy, physiology and neuropsychology of the frontal lobe*, second edition. New York, Raven Press, 1989.

40. Wu KK. Endothelial cells in hemostasis, thrombosis, and inflammation. *Hospital Practice* 27(4): 145-168, 1992.

41. Bench W, Friston KJ, Brown RG, Scott LC, Frackowiak RJJ, Dolan RJ. The anatomy of melancholia focal abnormalities of cerebral blood flow in major depression. *Psychol med* 22: 607-615, 1992.

42. Austin M-P, Dougall N, Ross M, Murray C, O'Carroll RE, Maffoot A, Embeier KP, Goodwin GM. Single phaton emission tomography with ^{99m}Tc = exametazine in major depression and the pattern of brain activity underlying the psychotic/neurotic continuum. *J Affect Dis* 26: 31-44, 1992.

43. Ichise M, Salit IE, Abbey SE, Chung D-G, Gray B, Kirsch JC, Freedman M. Assessment of regional cerebral perfusion by ^{99}Tc^{m}HMPAO SPECT in chronic fatigue syndrome. *Nuc Med Comm* 13: 767-772, 1992.

44. Neveu PJ. Asymmetrical brain modulation of the immune response. *Brain Res Rev* 17:101-107, 1992.

45. Mayberg HS, Robinson RS, Wong DF, et al. PET imaging of cortical S_2 serotonin receptors after stroke: lateralized changes relationship to depression. *Am J Psychiatry* 145(8): 937-943, 1988.

46. Prasher D, Findley L. Multi-modality sensory and auditory cognitive event-related potentials in myalgic encephalomyelitis and multiple sclerosis. In: Hyde, BM (ed.) *The Clinical and Scientific Basis of Myalgic Encephalomyelitis/ Chronic Fatigue Syndrome*. Ottawa: Nightingale Research Foundation, 1992.

47. Dager SR, Steen RG. Applications of magnetic resonance spectroscopy to the investigation of neuropsychiatric disorders. *Neuropsychopharmacology* 6(4): 249-263, 1992.

48. Iger LM. The MMPI as an aid to CFS diagnosis. *CFIDS Chronicle:* 35-38, Spring/Summer 1990.

49. Manu P, Lane TJ, Mathews DA. Somatization disorder in patients with chronic fatigue. *Psychosomatics* 30(4): 388-394,1989.

50. Glowa JR, Sternberg EW, Gold PW. Differential behavioral response in LEW/N and F344/N rats: effects of corticotropin releasing hormone. *Prog Neuropsychopharmacol Biol Psychiat* 16(4): 549-560, 1992.

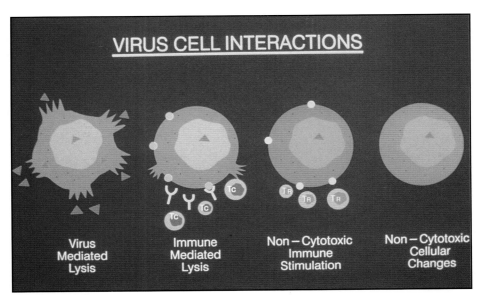

Physicians view viral diseases as killing or damaging cells. Viruses can cause only functional cellular impairment, by altering secretion of one or more transmitters, for example.

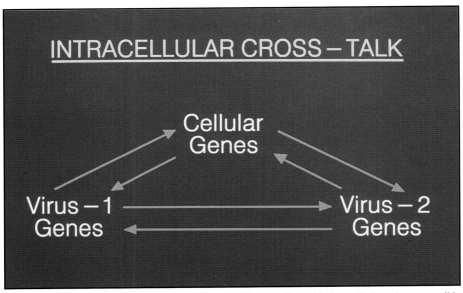

The gene products of a viral agent interact with host DNA, as well as with those of other viruses, possibly activating them, or making them more virulent ("transactivation").

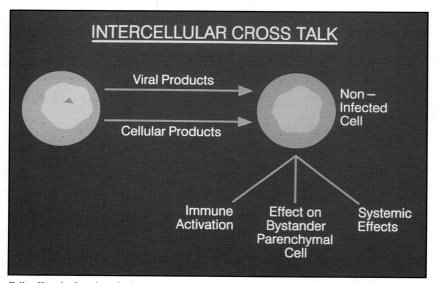

Cells affect the function of other cells, tissues, systems and the host by secreting products which act on adjacent cells, the local environment, or at a distance by transportation through blood or spinal fluid. Viral infections can alter the secretion of products normally made by the cell or can code for new products. These substances can cause uninfected cells to behave differently.

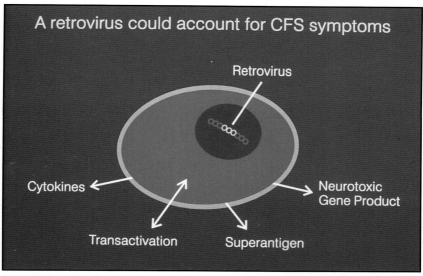

Although not necessary to produce the functional alterations of CFS, a retroviral agent could contribute to CFS pathophysiology. It could modulate production of cytokines, chemicals which alter the immune function of other cells. It could be transactivated by another virus, as has been proposed for HHV-6 and HIV, or even recombine with another viral agent such as a herpes virus. It could cause immune activation by coding for antigens that can bind to the variable region of the T-cell receptor, and could code for gene products which could be directly neurotoxic.

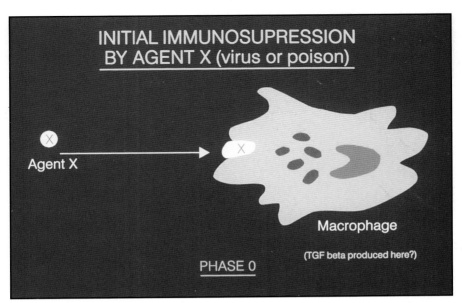

INITIAL IMMUNOSUPPRESSION BY AGENT X (virus or poison)

Agent X → Macrophage

(TGF beta produced here?)

PHASE 0

"Agent X," here depicted as a virus infecting a macrophage, could primarily infect other cells, including neurons, but exists in a latent state until activated by a triggering stimulus. "Agent X" could be a genetic predisposition, a psychological trauma affecting the developmental plasticity of the immature limbic system, an environmental toxin, or numerous other factors.

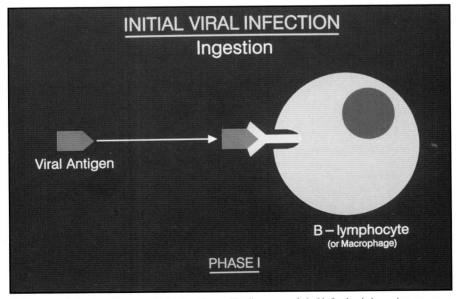

INITIAL VIRAL INFECTION Ingestion

Viral Antigen → B – lymphocyte (or Macrophage)

PHASE I

CFS commonly begins after an acute flu-like illness. The first stage of viral infection is *ingestion*, a process by which a virus enters a cell by mimicking a ligand for a specific receptor.

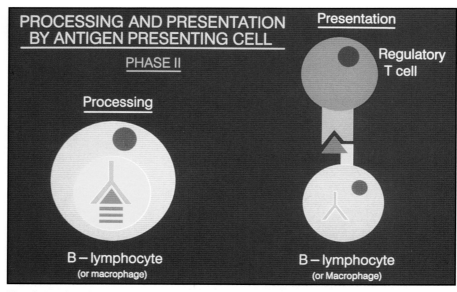

The viral antigen is digested into low molecular weight peptides ("processing") and then displayed ("presentation") to a regulatory T-cell by nesting in a highly individualized compartment, the Major Histocompatibility Complex (MHC). Efforts to alter the course of CFS with medications that affect processing and presentation have thus far been unsuccessful.

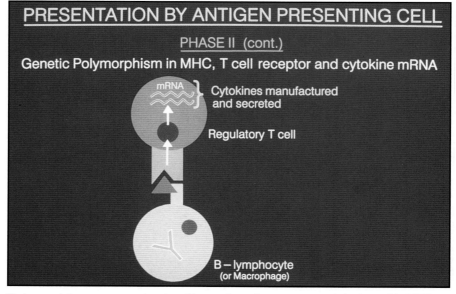

Each person's immune response is unique. The way that antigens are processed, the shape of the MHC and the T-cell receptor, and the amounts and kinds of cytokines that are manufactured in response to this interaction are all genetically regulated.

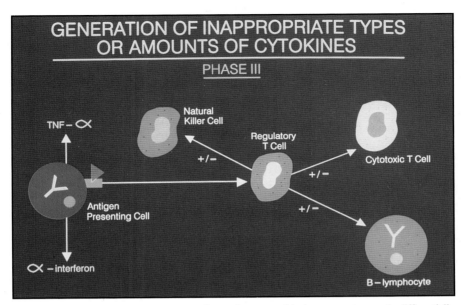

GENERATION OF INAPPROPRIATE TYPES OR AMOUNTS OF CYTOKINES

PHASE III

Depending upon the result of antigen presentation, various arms of the immune system can be differentially activated or suppressed. In CFS, we usually see decreased NK cell activity, increased cytotoxic T-cell activity, and increased B-cell antibody production, particularly for herpes viruses.

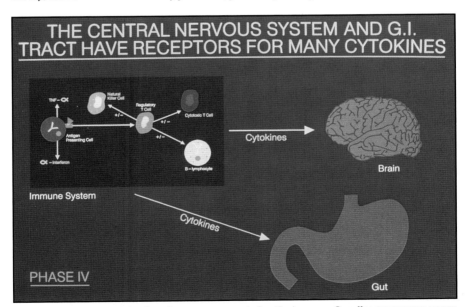

THE CENTRAL NERVOUS SYSTEM AND G.I. TRACT HAVE RECEPTORS FOR MANY CYTOKINES

PHASE IV

The immune system cannot be viewed as an autonomously functioning organ. Its cells act as sensory organs which closely monitor the internal milieu, communicating with other organs, particularly in the central nervous system, and altering their activity.

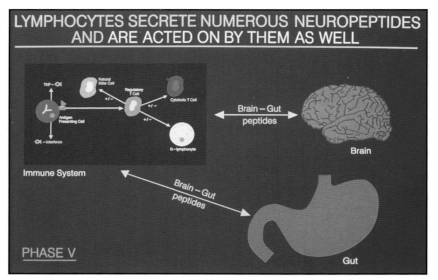

The central nervous system modulates the function of the immune system in a bidirectional manner, as well as regulating the function of other organ systems. Early workers in CFS tended to disregard the role of the brain in determining immune activity. Today we increasingly regard the body as a network of many types of transmitter substances which can comprise a "code" to exquisitely regulate neuronal structures depending upon the biochemical composition of the message.

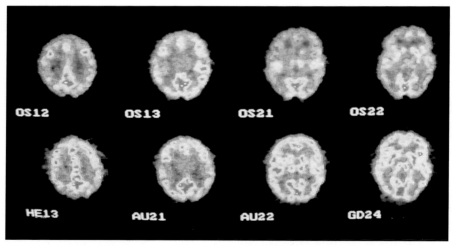

We have studied brain function in CFS in 3 ways. PET scan measures cerebral glucose utilization and blood flow. In these views, decreased glucose utilization is noted in the frontal lobes of the patient depicted superiorly as compared to a control subject.

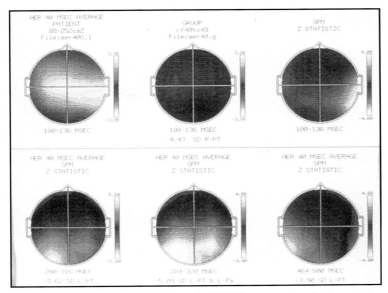

Topographic brain mapping in the form of a BEAM scan consistently demonstrates temporal lobe abnormalities, primarily in auditory and visual evoked responses. A normal BEAM scan should be completely symmetrical.

CFIDS (N=100)	Eyes Closed Spectral Average	Eyes Open Spectral Average	Long Latency Visual Evoked Response	Long Latency Auditory Evoked Response
Left Frontal	11	7	11	18
Right Frontal	7	2	7	15
Left Anterior Temporal	16	5	48	59
Right Anterior Temporal	7	2	8	25
Left Mid – Temporal	18	10	75	87
Right Mid – Temporal	6	2	27	25
Left Posterior Temporal	23	15	67	88
Right Posterior Temporal	6	6	23	37
Left Occipital	6	5	16	42
Right Occipital	2	3	12	27
Left Mid – Central	6	7	17	31
Right Mid – Central	1	1	8	21
Left Parietal	5	6	17	33
Right Parietal	1	1	6	22

Other brain areas are also abnormal in BEAM recordings, but temporal lobe abnormalities predominate.

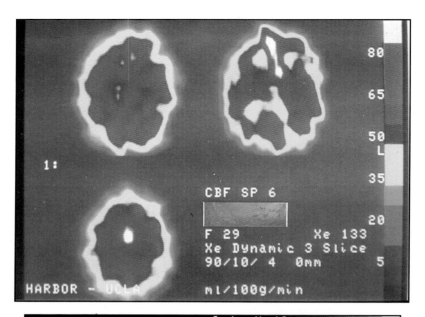

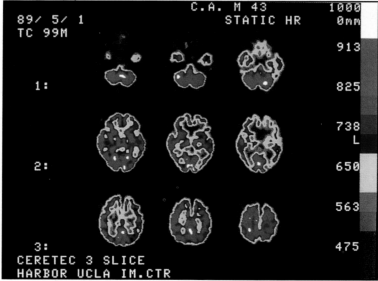

SPECT scanning of the brain measures regional cerebral blood flow. In the system discussed in this book, [133]Xenon and technetium HMPAO are used as radioisotopes to image blood flow. Normal [133]Xenon and HMPAO scans are shown.

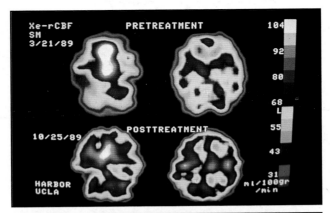

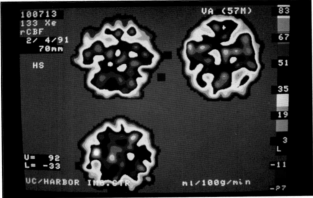

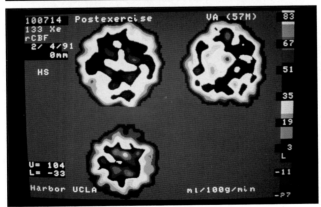

Resting brain SPECT scans done with HMPAO distinguish CFS patients from normals and those with depression and medical diseases, but assessing function with ^{133}Xenon pre- and post-exercise usually reveals a pronounced worsening of hypoperfusion after exercising, often persisting until the next day. We are still assessing the response of comparison groups in this paradigm. Brain perfusion improves after successful treatment.

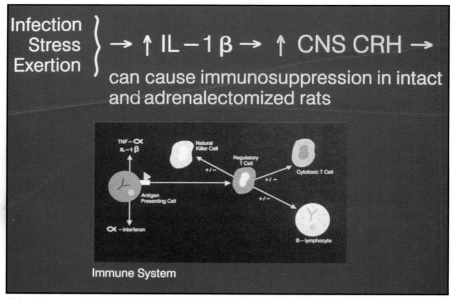

Infection ⎫
Stress   ⎬ → ↑ IL − 1β → ↑ CNS CRH →
Exertion ⎭

can cause immunosuppression in intact and adrenalectomized rats

Immune System

Although some assign the central role in the regulation of homeostasis to corticotropin releasing hormone (CRH), regulation of such functions as blood flow and sleep do not seem to involve CRH as its role is currently understood. A more integrative substance is central interleukin-1 beta (IL-1 beta), which stimulates CRH with resultant immunosuppression.

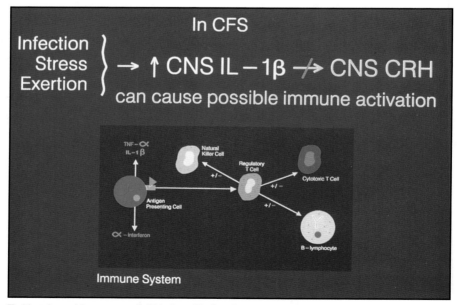

In CFS

Infection ⎫
Stress   ⎬ → ↑ CNS IL − 1β ↛ CNS CRH
Exertion ⎭

can cause possible immune activation

Immune System

IL-1 beta is sensitive to stress of all kinds, and its function can be modulated by many other centrally active substances, especially cytokines which are independently regulated from IL-1. Decreased central action of IL-1 beta and CRH, possibly occurring in CFS, could result in peripheral immune activation.

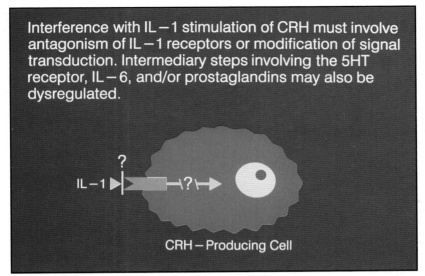

Interference with IL-1 stimulation of CRH must involve antagonism of IL-1 receptors or modification of signal transduction. Intermediary steps involving the 5HT receptor, IL-6, and/or prostaglandins may also be dysregulated.

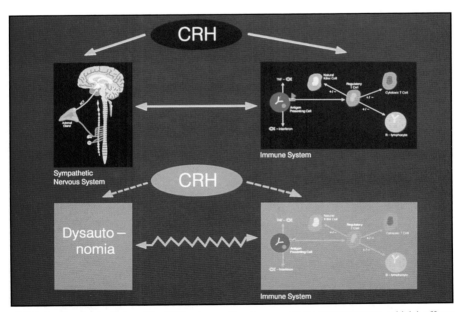

CRH is involved in regulation of the HPA axis as well as the sympathetic nervous system, which it affects independent of adrenocortical activity by circulating through the neuraxis. Decreased activity of CRH would affect the activity of both systems, which also directly influence each other.

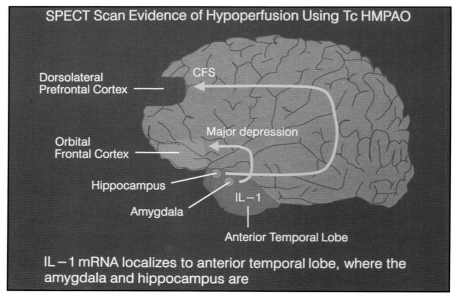

SPECT Scan Evidence of Hypoperfusion Using Tc HMPAO

Dorsolateral
Prefrontal Cortex ——

CFS

Orbital
Frontal Cortex ——

Major depression

Hippocampus

Amygdala

IL – 1

Anterior Temporal Lobe

IL – 1 mRNA localizes to anterior temporal lobe, where the amygdala and hippocampus are

SPECT scans in CFS show anterior temporal and dorsolateral prefrontal hypoperfusion, predominantly in the right hemisphere. The hippocampus is thought to regulate the dorsolateral prefrontal cortex, and the hippocampus is one of the few places in the brain where IL-1 beta mRNA is found.

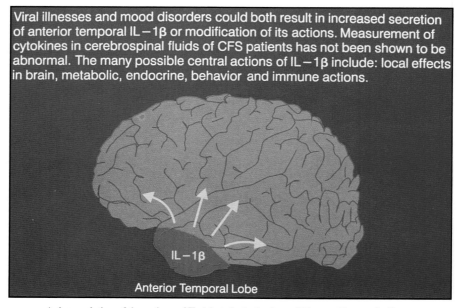

Viral illnesses and mood disorders could both result in increased secretion of anterior temporal IL – 1β or modification of its actions. Measurement of cytokines in cerebrospinal fluids of CFS patients has not been shown to be abnormal. The many possible central actions of IL – 1β include: local effects in brain, metabolic, endocrine, behavior and immune actions.

IL – 1β

Anterior Temporal Lobe

A dysregulation of the actions of IL-1 beta in the brain could have widespread effects.

Actions Of IL–1 In The Brain

1) **Local Effects In Brain:** altered EEG and neuronal activity, inhibition of long term potentiation, cortical inhibitory postsynaptic function, neurotransmitter release / turnover, induction of NGF, self–induction (of IL–1β), astrogliosis, neovascularization and augmentation of $GABA_A$ receptor function.

2) **Metabolic Actions:** fever, increased metabolic rate (thermogenesis), sympathetic activation of brown fat, hypophagia, and altered gastric function.

3) **Endocrine Actions:** hypothalamic–pituitary hormone release (CRH, GnRH, TSH, ACTH), pituitary–adrenal activation and insulin release.

4) **Behavioral Actions:** sleep, and sickness behavior (e.g., reduced exploration), hypalgesia.

5) **Immune Actions:** peripheral IL–6 release, decreased peripheral IL–2 production, reduced natural killer cell activity, leukocytosis, and hepatic acute phase protein synthesis.

Central actions of IL-1 beta (after NJ Rothwell) which appear to be important in CFS include its action on the $GABA_A$ receptor (anxiety, PMS), thermogenesis (low temperature and inability to appropriately elevate it, weight gain), sleep disorders (IL-1 is involved in sleep induction), pain (central IL-1 is hypalgesic), regulation of the autonomic nervous system (low blood pressure, Raynaud's disorder), and of numerous hormones and transmitter substances (serotonin, various neuropeptides, prostaglandins, and others).

ANTAGONIZING IL-1

IL-1ra

IL-1 RtI antibodies

Soluble IL-R proteins

TGF-beta ($\downarrow$ IL-1R expression)

IFN gamma

retroviral envelope protein (p15E)

alpha MSH and Ly-Pro-Val

CRH

methyl ester muramyl dipeptide

IL-4

IL-10

Numerous substances can inhibit the action of IL-1 beta. They include IL-1ra, TGF-beta, and IL-10. IL-4 is not a good candidate because it decreases production of IL-1.

Cytokine levels in serum and cerebrospinal fluid in patients with chronic fatigue syndrome (CFS) and control subjects.		
	Group		
Cytokine, sample	CFS (n = 25)	Myelography (n = 28)	CNS infections (n = 10)
IFN-α			
Serum	0.5 (0.9)	0.6 (0.9)	7.5 (4.7)
CSF	3.3 (0.5)*	2.9 (0.7)*	5.5 (3.3)
IFN-γ			
Serum	0	0	0
CSF	0	0	1.4 (1.9)
Neopterin			
Serum	6.7 (4.0)	11 (6.3)	—
CSF	2.9 (3.0)	3.1 (1.7)	—
IL-1β			
Serum	17.1 (4.4)	17.7 (5.5)	—
CSF	20.5 (4.1)	20.5 (4.1)	—
TNFα			
Serum	10.0 (2.6)	9.7 (1.6)	9.1 (2.2)
CSF	5.0 (7.6)	4.1 (0.9)	11.5 (12.1)

Measurement of CSF cytokines in CFS patients by Lloyd et al. do not show a decreased concentration of IL-1 beta, so if this cytokine is involved in pathogenesis, there must be interference with its actions.

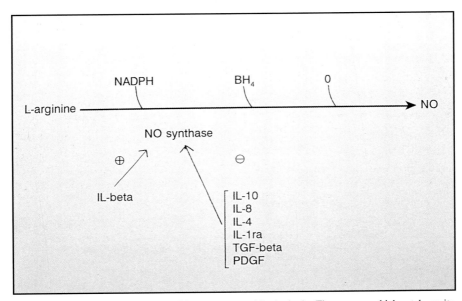

Nitric oxide may be the primary vasodilatory compound in the body. The enzyme which catalyzes its synthesis, nitric oxide (NO) synthase, is probably constitutively stimulated by IL-1 to antagonize vasospasm. NO synthase may be antagonized by some of the same cytokines which inhibit the action of IL-1. The vasoconstriction that is seen on CFS SPECT scans may thus be a result of IL-1 antagonism.

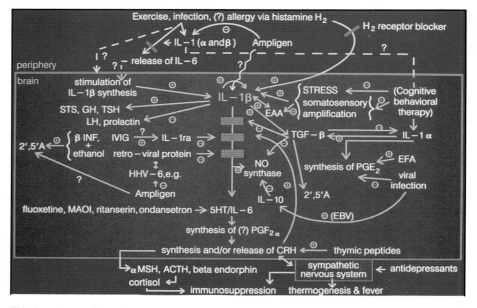

This flow diagram is used as a model for possible dysfunctional CNS neuroregulatory pathways in CFS. Stemming from the clinical observation that virtually any type of stress (exercise, emotional, cognitive, infectious, sleep deprivation) makes CFS worse, it postulates that the pleotropic cytokine interleukin-1 beta (IL-1ß) has a central role in maintaining homeostasis.

Through intermediaries such as 5HT, IL-6, and prostaglandins (PG), central IL-1ß stimulates, modulates, or inhibits the release of numerous neuropeptides and other transmitter substances, and is known to be involved in sleep induction, immunosuppression, hypalgesia, fever, thermogenesis, and weight loss through activation of brown fat. Many of its effects occur as a result of increased corticotropin releasing hormone (CRH) production. Other important functions of IL-1ß include stimulation of nitric oxide synthase to promote vasodilation and facilitation of opening of the chloride channel of the GABA receptor.

The neuroanatomic localization of IL-1 mRNA in the dentate gyrus and the dorsal raphe suggests functional results of antagonism of IL-1 effect by various endogenous substances such as transforming growth factor beta (TGF-ß), IL-10, an independently regulated cytokine called IL-1ra (receptor antagonist), and viral protein gene products which can interfere with IL-1ß signal transduction.

Sudden state changes could be transduced by excitatory amino acids (EAA's). Intero- and exteroceptive stimuli, integrated in paralimbic areas, could undergo faulty processing if a multifactorial limbic encephalopathy producing increased synaptogenesis were present, resulting in somatosensory amplification. Such dysfunction is amenable to cognitive behavioral therapy.

This model predicts that CFS patients would have decreased central biogenic amines, and that production of substances such as cortisol, growth hormone, beta endorphin, and catecholamines after a stress such as exercise would be impaired. It should be difficult to induce fever in this population and such patients should not increase, and may even reduce, regional cerebral blood flow after exercise. Anxiety, sleep, weight gain, low blood pressure, and pain disorders should be more prevalent in this population, which may have peripheral immune activation as a result of impaired central immunosuppression.

Although tremendously oversimplified, the model that CFS symptoms are caused by an imbalance between IL-1 beta and its endogenous or multifactorially induced inhibitors can enhance understanding of the disorder and direct efforts toward remediation.

See text for further details.

Treatment of Chronic Fatigue Syndrome

SUMMARY. Almost all chronic fatigue syndrome treatment is in an experimental stage, and some physicians are reluctant to engage in treatment protocols that have not had rigorous experimental trials. CFS patients are difficult to manage, since they present long lists of symptoms, extensive histories, and may require extended follow-up. Various other problems include limit-setting for therapy, insurance difficulties, and applying treatments which are based on anecdotal clinical success shared through professional networking. When viewing CFS as a multicausal limbic encephalopathy in a dysregulated neuroimmune network, the physician can apply a number of therapeutic interventions: anti-infective, immunomodulatory, neuroendocrine, neuropharmacologic, neurobehavioral, symptom-oriented, and "other." Several viruses have been detected by the Polymerase Chain Reaction (PCR): CMV, Epstein-Barr, and HHV-6 have all been detected in CFS patients in this manner. Therapeutic interventions used for subsets of CFS include antibiotics, anti-virals, immunomodulatory agents, interferon, H-2 blockers, intravenous immunoglobulin (IVIG), kutapressin, oral alpha interferon, NSAIDS, and many psychotropic medications. The latter include benzodiazepines, tricyclic antidepressants, monoamine oxidase inhibitors, and fluoxetine. The recent discovery of nitric oxide as a neurotransmitter, as well as a vasodilator, has broken new treatment ground in CFS, and using nitroglycerin as a source of nitric oxide produced symptom relief when other medications have failed. In addition, a large number of patients have already tried alternative medications with the cooperation of their contacts in the AIDS underground.

[DocuSerial™ co-indexing entry]

"Treatment of Chronic Fatigue Syndrome," Goldstein, J.A. Published in: *Haworth Library of the Medical Neurobiology of Somatic Disorders* (The Haworth Medical Press), Volume 1, 1993 and *Chronic Fatigue Syndromes: The Limbic Hypothesis*, Goldstein, J.A., The Haworth Medical Press, 1993.

Virtually all CFS treatment can be termed experimental, thus if going by practice guidelines which state that no experimental therapy may be given for any condition unless under protocol, then CFS should not be treated. Many physicians adhere to this principle and tell patients to go home and rest until they feel better, or words to that effect. In truth, many CFS patients are difficult to treat. There is no effective standard therapy, and there is a multiplicity of complaints which often must be addressed individually, since a specific underlying cause cannot be dealt with at present. Physicians are allowed at their discretion to prescribe FDA-approved drugs for non-FDA recommended purposes when the individual patient's needs justify such use.

Some CFS patients are very descriptive of how they feel, and the time required to obtain a complete history is lengthy. In conducting a CFS practice, I have had to double the amount of time I allot for new patients and follow-up visits, and often this extension is not sufficient. It is not unusual for a follow-up visit to last one hour in my office, and longer if the amount of time spent doing reports and filling out forms is factored in. I commonly spend three hours a day returning patient phone calls, some of which are lengthy. It is difficult to bill insurance for this time, or for comprehensive office visits on every patient encounter, although the time spent justifies this insurance code.

The physician must be alert for the CFS patient with borderline personality or a related severe "character" disorder. Most practices can handle only two or three such patients at one time, but borderline personality, which is probably a limbic disorder, seems to be overrepresented in the CFS population, even though this diagnosis still applies to a small minority of CFS patients. A borderline patient may demonstrate lability of affect, idealization and denigration of his physician, and intense anger. Suicidal behavior is common. These traits are seen in chronic illness to a certain extent, but are greatly magnified with the borderline CFS patient.

It is also difficult to be limit-setting, as one must be with personality disorder patients, and at the same time investigative in trying new treatment approaches. The best way to manage such patients is to have them seen concurrently by a psychotherapist, but such a policy is difficult to enforce when the patient is not able to afford psychotherapy or is resistant to entering therapy.

The situation is made more difficult by the refusal of some insurers to pay a claim when the patient has been diagnosed with CFS, and by the fact that many patients have lost their insurance because they are unable to work. Large HMOs will often not diagnose CFS. Sometimes this refusal appears to be on the basis of conservatism. Other times it appears to be a fiscally motivated policy since (understandably), HMO physicians cannot spend 90 to 120 minutes on each initial consultation, 30 to 60 minutes on a follow-up, or consider ordering esoteric tests and non-standard treatments.

Much of the problem has to do with ambiguity in the evaluation and treatment process. Even I, who rather enjoy applying different pathophysiologic paradigms to difficult clinical situations, sometimes long for the cut-and-dried patient encounters that dermatologists and orthopedists often have, not to mention their long vacations. If one is looking for certainty, the physician will not find it in a CFS practice.

DETERMINING PATHOPHYSIOLOGY

Before a treatment can be prescribed, a pathophysiology must be assigned. The treatment approaches in CFS are determined by whether a physician views the disorder as a viral illness with immune dysfunction or a psychiatric problem. Although there appear to be two camps presently, many physicians are trying to reach a middle ground, and some take a different approach. These orientations are quite diverse and include nutritional medicine, antiparasitic and anti-candidal approaches, environmental medicine and clinical ecology, antioxidant orientation, acupuncture, chiropractic, altering brain and body electromagnetism, live cell therapy, naturopathy, homeopathy, Eastern and Ayurvedic medicine, and others too numerous to mention. It is helpful for the CFS physician to be acquainted with alternative medicine, since his patients often will be, and to resist labeling something "quackery" just because it does not make sense to him. Treatment is still a contract between physician and patient, and the approach taken depends on the orientation of the physician and his willingness to explore new avenues with the informed consent of the patient, although sometimes the patient will have his or her own novel suggestions. It is certainly ethical for a physician to believe that he is serving a patient's interest best by not deviating from standard CFS treatment (which is no treatment). Some physicians believe that the only treatments prescribed should be those proven effective by multiple double-blind experiments. It should also be ethical to try any treatment for which there appears to be a scientific rationale and a favorable risk/benefit ratio. Since there have been only two treatments for CFS with published results of double-blind experiments, it is difficult to choose among alternatives.

Two double-blind studies of high-dose IV immunoglobulin (higher than most physicians use for CFS) reached opposite conclusions regarding efficacy.[1,2] One is left with few objective guidelines.

Viewing CFS as a multicausal limbic encephalopathy in a dysregulated neuroimmune network enables the physician to generate pathophysiologic hypotheses which lend themselves to rational therapeutic intervention. They can be divided into:

1. Anti-infective
2. Immunomodulatory
3. Neuroendocrine
4. Neuropharmacologic
5. Neurobehavioral
6. Symptom-oriented, and
7. "Other."

Anti-Infective Intervention

Several viruses have been detected by polymerase chain reaction (PCR) and fewer by culture in a significantly higher percentage than in normal controls. CMV, Epstein-Barr virus, and HHV-6 have all been detected by PCR. Whether these viruses should be treated or not is uncertain. It is well known that CMV is found in normal individuals and does not cause target organ damage. Whether these viruses cause transactivation of another infectious agent such as a retrovirus or interact with the host genome to alter cell function in CFS is undecided. My approach would be to treat an infected patient with antiviral chemotherapy if a relatively nontoxic agent could be used against a virus which had some sensitivity. The only agent I could use at this time is acyclovir, which is safe when used appropriately in high doses. It has some effect against EB virus. I do not believe a good risk/benefit ratio exists for using agents such as ganciclovir or foscarnet although I have heard of their use by certain clinicians when PCR's were positive for the appropriate viruses. I would look forward to seeing the results of such interventions. Perhaps evidence of immune activation would constitute some grounds for intervention, as well as abnormalities in brain functional imaging and/or neuropsychological testing, indicating a viral encephalopathy. If the virus were detected in the CSF, even in the absence of an immune response such as a lymphocytosis, antiviral chemotherapy could be justified in difficult cases. Remember that viruses can alter cellular function without changing morphology or causing cell death. Getting insurance companies to pay for this sort of treatment, which is initially done in hospital, is difficult. Should the time for infusion be prolonged, permanent catheter placement would be necessary so that chemotherapy could be conducted at home. It is only very recently that PCRs for the herpesviruses have become available to the clinician.

As of this writing, we are evaluating antiviral agents in the hope of finding one to be used in culture-positive patients in an experimental protocol. Ampligen is being tested currently, and has been reported to be effective in vitro against HHV-6, demonstrating that it has antiviral properties as well as immunomodulatory ones. I know of no drugs useful against enteroviruses.

Some patients with a clinical picture that looks very much like CFS have been treated with ceftriaxone (Rocephin) because they had positive repeat antibody titers to *borrelia burgdorferi*. A few of these patients report a good response, although not a cure. Before I use this treatment more often I would like to see a PCR for *b. burgdorferi* become available. Two grams of ceftriaxone a day for two weeks is expensive, but not outlandishly so, and the treatment is safe. I will use it in the treatment-resistant patient but prefer to get an infectious disease consultation first.

Very few of my patients have responded to a low sugar diet and fluconazole (Diflucan), but those who did had a dramatic improvement. My experience differs from that reported by Dr. Carol Jessop, who treats many of her CFS patients this way. I have not had good results with these agents. Our outcomes may differ because I use anticandidal therapy late in treatment trials while she does it early in the course. Dr. Jessop believes that candidiasis may be a primary cause of CFS perhaps as a result of prolonged antibiotic use as well as a secondary colonizer due to a T-cell dysfunction caused by CFS.[3]

Numerous antiparasitic drugs are used, both prescription and non-prescription, to treat a wide variety of organisms, of which giardia is the most common. I diagnose intestinal parasites infrequently, and have generally used metronidazole to treat giardiasis. Parasites may be acquired from foreign travel or from infected workers in the United States who have come from developing countries.[4]

Alterations in the intestinal microflora have also been implicated in the pathogenesis of CFS. It is difficult to kill the bad bacteria without killing the good ones also, and efforts to repopulate the microflora with exotic remedies such as capsules of dung have not been notably effective to my knowledge. There is a strong gut-brain connection in CFS and these measures may have value in selected patients, but further investigation is necessary before I could recommend such an approach.

If a patient has CFS caused by an existing infection, i.e., not a "post-infectious" fatigue syndrome, it could be worsened by almost any secondary infection, whether viral, bacterial, rickettsial, mycoplasmal, fungal, chlamydial, or what have you. Any infectious agent alters the immune status of the host and also resistance to current infections. If the host immune status is altered, certain infections, either from latent or exogenous microbial origin, may occur. Infections may also increase the production of cytokines as the immune system is activated in response to the invader.

Some of my patients feel better for no apparent reason when they take antibiotics. The response could, of course, be a placebo effect, since "antibiotic" still has a "wonder drug" connotation to many. Other possibilities are that there is an undiagnosed infection, perhaps in the sinuses, that could be contributing to fatigue, or that the antibiotics are instead working as immunomodulators. Many antibiotics have this property to some extent.

Agents that would block the receptors for virus penetration into a cell much in the manner in which peptide T blocks the HIV gp120 and the CD4 receptor protein might be feasible. The limbic system has receptors which have been mapped by monoclonal antibodies.[5] There is a paraneoplastic syndrome, "limbic encephalitis," in which a patient develops an inflammatory infiltrate in limbic structures in association with a neoplasm.[6] A common virus, HSV-1, has a tropism for receptors in the medial temporal lobe where it can cause a subclinical infection which could lead to temporolimbic epilepsy.[7] Borna virus can cause a limbic encephalitis in animals and perhaps humans.[8] Antibodies to Borna virus have been detected in some patients with affective disorders, but not in controls.[9] The spread of a murine neurotropic coronavirus through the olfactory pathway into the limbic system has been demonstrated.[10] Viruses that infect neurons may also enter lymphocytes, since both types of cells share receptors to a great degree.

The psychiatrists working in CFS research have not addressed the issue of a viral cause for behavioral alteration, although there is an occasional allusion to the effect of cytokines. Since the work of M. Oldstone and colleagues has demonstrated that a viral infection of a neuron can alter the secretion of a single neurotransmitter as its only metabolic perturbation,[11] the possible effects of viral CNS infections are virtually unlimited. These effects can persist after the viral infection has been eliminated, thus establishing a rational mechanism for post-viral syndromes. The notion of treating many neurobehavioral disorders with antimicrobial agents is an exciting one. The ameliorative effect of zidovudine on the HIV-1-associated cognitive/motor complex may be just a harbinger of what is to come.

Immunomodulatory Intervention

Immunomodulatory agents offer great promise. Most cytokines have more than one effect, depending on the cell type that has the appropriate receptors. It has been suggested that the main reason for the existence of the blood-brain barrier is to segregate transmitters manufactured in the brain from those in the periphery, since the transmitters are the same. Although my experience using immuno-suppressive agents in CFS has not been good, it may be that I have just not chosen the right drugs. Azathioprine, cyclophosphamide, and methotrexate, used in low doses as for rheumatoid arthritis or multiple sclerosis, did not help any of my patients when I tried them a few years ago; I did not use cyclosporin. This drug has a more specific effect on T-lymphocyte activation, particularly blocking interleukin-2 and its receptor, and also IL-1, IL-3, IL-4, and gamma interferon. It is not effective in MS. As we learn more about the nature of lymphocyte activation in CFS, the use of immunosuppres-sive agents in selected patients might be feasible.

A suggestion about why immunosuppressive drugs might be use-ful in CFS comes from their use in experimental models of drug withdrawal. Cyclosporin has been shown to ameliorate opioid absti-nence syndrome.[12,13] The mechanism of action is unclear, since increased levels of IL-1, for example, are associated with elevation of CRH and subsequent stimulation of proopiomelanocortin secre-tion, producing ACTH and beta endorphin. Increased activity of $GABA_A$ receptors are also associated with IL-1 secretion. Gluco-corticoids exert feedback inhibition of IL-1 synthesis and actions. IL-1 beta also stimulates serotonin production. It would thus appear that agents which lower IL-1 levels (and presumably IL-2 levels as well) would produce anxiety and worsen abstinence syndromes. There must be one or more intermediary transmitters that are not being considered, since if CRH hyposecretion is associated with CFS, it must also be related to some cases of panic disorder. I can only conjecture how cyclosporin would work in panic disorder, since agents to attenuate opioid withdrawal act either at the opioid or alpha-2 adrenergic receptor. It is effective, however, in athymic ("nude") mice and thus must have a direct central effect, probably in the limbic system. Anterior cingulotomy for intractable pain abolishes withdrawal symptoms in drug-dependent patients.[14]

Little is yet known about the interface of the cytokines with the neuropeptides in the brain. Although IL-1 may stimulate CRH, it may instead (or also) act at the pituitary level to increase ACTH secretion. CRH has been shown to upregulate IL-1 receptors in mouse AtT-20 pituitary tumor cells.[15] Short-term administration of interferon alpha-2 in therapeutic doses to patients with chronic hepatitis B produced rises in cortisol and ACTH to over 300% of baseline. The actions were related to side effects like fever or other flu-like symptoms.[16] IL-2 and gamma interferon have also been shown to stimulate the secretion of cortisol in man.

Interferon alpha-2 does not cross the blood-brain barrier well, and elevations in ACTH and cortisol were not directly related to serum interferon alpha-2 levels. Induction of ACTH secretion by lymphocytes was considered unlikely. Some lymphocytes may have CRH activity, but CRH does not enter the brain easily, either. It can, however, have a pro-inflammatory effect in the periphery.

It has been suggested that CFS is a cytokine-mediated illness, at least in some patients. Some cellular enzyme measurements would suggest increased production of interferons as well as interleukins. One of these systems, induced by interferon, is 2′5′-oligo A synthetase/RNaseL.[17] This system exerts its antiviral effect by enzymatically degrading viral RNA, thereby reducing its availability as a template for translocation into viral proteins. The enzyme is upregulated by viral double-stranded RNA and converts viral RNA into "specific cleavage products." In the process, it uses up large amounts of cellular ATP and digests cellular RNA as well. This rapid catabolism of ATP may contribute to the fatigue and cognitive dysfunction that CFS patients feel, and since 2,5A levels are very high in some CFS patients, the cause of the fatigue in these individuals could possibly be different than in those with normal 2,5A levels. Treatment with Ampligen in these cases may improve CFS symptoms without having an effect on characterologic depression, although reactive depression should improve. The drug must be given intravenously two or three times a week. Unfortunately, many patients relapse, or even rebound, when the drug is discontinued.

I start most of my patients on H-2 blockers, usually ranitidine (Zantac), 150 mg BID. Other H-2 blockers are less effective, but may be tried when ranitidine is not well tolerated. Lymphocytes and neurons have H-2 receptors. CD8 cells may secrete less supressor factors if the H-2 receptor is blocked. H-2 blockers may exert their anti-ulcer effects by binding to receptors on gastric immunocytes.[18] There is a high density of H-2 receptors in the brain, particularly in the neocortex and hippocampus. Several studies indicate that different subclasses of H-2 receptors are expressed on a single cell, probably accounting for the differential response. H-2 receptor agonists are neuronal inhibitors; thus, antagonists could be activators. A dysregulation of H-2 receptors may exist in about 20% of CFS patients who appear to respond to ranitidine. A small proportion become agitated or "hyper," and are not able to tolerate the medication. This adverse reaction occurs often enough in CFS patients for me to warn them of it. Some are not able to tolerate ranitidine for this reason. It is thought by some that H-2 blockers increase CRH levels. The H-1 and the H-2 receptors are increasingly being recognized as being important in cytokine regulation.[19] Cytokines, thought to play an endocrine function, have been found to be increased in acute infectious mononucleosis, although not in CFS.[20] I have found cimetidine and ranitidine extremely effective in rapidly eliminating the symptoms of acute mononucleosis.

Intravenous immunoglobulin (IVIG) is quite helpful to certain patients. It is used in disorders of T-cell activation and was employed in a high dose in a double-blind Australian study which regarded CFS as a disorder of excessive cytokine production which may occur in genetically predisposed individuals after antigenic stimulation. Forty-three percent of study participants had a beneficial response.[21]

IVIG has been used successfully in immunologically mediated neurologic disorders, and also in intractable epilepsy of childhood, in which no immunologic abnormality can be demonstrated.[22] Some of my CFS patients get hypomanic after IVIG, and this treatment has precipitated an acute manic episode in two fatigued bipolar patients of mine. Currently I give 5 gm IVIG weekly, or 10 gm every other week until a total dose of 60 gm is reached. A patient may not have a good response until this level is attained, although most will not be able to continue to pay for a treatment that might not work. Most insurance companies will not reimburse for IVIG treatment of CFS. Alternative ways that IVIG might work in CFS would be by binding to cytokines and inactivating them (CNS IL-1ra), by an antiidiotypic effect on neuronal autoantibodies, (which are not present in CFS), by solubilizing immune complexes (common in CFS), although their role in pathogenesis is uncertain, and by down-regulation of Fc receptors so that immune complexes cannot be formed. IVIG may also increase levels of CD8+ suppressor T-cells.[23] The Fc part of immunoglobulins has been shown to bind to pituitary ACTH-producing cells.[24] Levels of serum immunoglobulins or IgG subclasses do not predict IVIG response in CFS, nor does, unfortunately, evidence of immune activation. The Australian group did suggest that decreased levels of CD4 cells might be associated with a beneficial result.

Kutapressin is a porcine liver extract of low molecular weight peptides which are thought to have an immunomodulatory action, since results on a test of mitogen stimulation, the single lymphocyte immune function, improve if initially suppressed. Kutapressin is given by intramuscular injection. Results have been excellent as reported in open trials by experimenters from Houston.[25] Many of us do not find the response to be nearly that good, and some CFS clinicians have stopped using it altogether. Active peptides from the parent Kutapressin have been isolated. This presumably more potent biological response modifier will be starting clinical trials shortly.

There are a number of other immunomodulatory compounds which have helped a few of my patients or that I think show promise. These include lentinan and LEM, lentinan being a single glucan from *Lentinus edodes,* the Shiitake mushroom, and LEM being a mixture of various glucans. Suzuki and co-workers in Japan have used lentinan IV in low natural killer cell syndrome (LNKS), which may be similar to CFS. Lentinan elevated interferon levels acutely and then increased NK cell activity.[26] LEM is given orally.

Thymic hormones, not too useful in AIDS, might be helpful in CFS, in which T-cell dysfunction is not as severe. Most immunomodulatory treatments for AIDS work better if combined with antiviral agents. Certain thymic fractions may have neuropeptide agonist properties. The partial purified thymic preparation TP5 was potent in stimulating CRH secretion in rat whole medial basal hypothalamic explants.[27]

Transfer factor, a leukocyte dialysate, has been used by several groups. The only double-blind study was done by the Australians who found no efficacy.[28] It is claimed by those who still use it that the Australian transfer factor was made improperly. Using disease-specific transfer factor made from household contacts is thought to be important.

Isoprinosine potentiates mitogen proliferation, IL-2 production, macrophage chemotaxis, and natural killer cell activity. It may also be thymomimetic and enhance gamma interferon production. It has few adverse reactions. It can increase uric acid levels. Some of my patients have reported improvement, but not impressively. Two developed gout. It has been suggested that isoprinosine may have optimum effectiveness in CFS when administered for only three consecutive days per week.[29]

DTC, or Imuthiol, is a medication that showed some promise in CFS, but the pharmaceutical company that manufactures it has suspended trials. The FDA denied a treatment IND (investigational new drug protocol) for expanded use in AIDS in 1990. The drug, which has few side effects except Antabuse-like reactions, has thymomimetic effects and apparently has some benefit. Levamisole has effects similar to DTC on immunomodulation by the neocortex. Imuthiol is thought to aid in the replacement of T-cell regulatory factors. Renoux and Renoux find that left cortical injury inhibits T-cell and NK cell function, and that the right cortex inhibits the activating effect of the left cortex.[30] Could right cortical inhibitory function be related to a lateralization of function of IL-1 beta?

DHEA, dehydroepiandrosterone, is an adrenal androgen with numerous purported immunomodulatory and stimulatory effects. It has been reported to treat obesity, stress, aging, and cancer. DHEA is the adrenal steroid produced in the highest quantity, yet it has no function recognized by the medical community. DHEA sulfate is measured in the diagnosis of hirsutism. Some of my patients have obtained DHEA from buyers' clubs and report more energy. Others had no improvement. Although I do not prescribe it, my impression is that it has limited efficacy. Other researchers disagree.[31] The concentration of DHEA in serum suggests it must have biologic activity. It is also regulated independently of ACTH.[32] Some CFS patients have very low levels of DHEA sulfate.

Substances such as DHEA and the first compound after cholesterol in steroid biosynthesis, pregnenolone, are called "neurosteroids" or neurally active steroids. They appear to be endogenous modulators of GABA-stimulated chloride ion conductance.[33] Neurosteroids have been shown to be positive and negative allosteric effectors of the GABA$_A$ receptor complex.

Naturally occurring 3-alpha-hydroxy ring A-reduced metabolites of progesterone and deoxycorticosterone have been shown to act as positive allosteric modulators of GABA-gated chloride ion conductance,[34] and are 1000 times more potent at this receptor than pentobarbital. Neurosteroids seem to act at a different site than barbiturates and benzodiazepines. Adrenalcorticoids or progesterone do not have this effect unless they are metabolized to a 3-alpha-hydroxyl derivative. GABA$_A$ receptors in the frontal cortex are extremely sensitive to the effects of neurosteroids, which apparently can be synthesized by glial cells in the brain.[35]

Negative allosteric modulators of GABA-gated chloride ion conductance include pregnenolone and DHEA. The brain has higher levels of these compounds than any other organ, and brain concentrations are independent of production peripherally.[36] Some neurosteroids appear to have anxiolytic properties in animals.[37] Neurosteroids have considerable potential in treating CFS and related disorders such as premenstrual syndrome, anxiety disorders, fibromyalgia, and sleep disorders.

Low-dose oral alpha interferon produces mild to moderate symptomatic improvement in some patients. Oral interferon in a dose of 200 units is now distributed in the form of a tablet which is held in the mouth until it dissolves. Interferon in such a low dose could interact with receptors in the oropharynx which connect to the limbic system and may even be directly transported there.[38] Oral alpha interferon is unlikely to directly activate antiviral systems in infected cells. Some clinicians believe that Kutapressin and low dose oral alpha interferon have a synergistic effect.

A combination of gamma linoleic acid (GLA) and eicosapentanoic acid (EPA), essential fatty acids, worked better than a placebo in a double-blind British study, in which better effects were shown after fifteen weeks than after five.[39] Viral infections are thought to block delta-6 desaturase, an enzyme which converts linoleic into gamma linoleic acid. The most impressive result was in reduction of palpitations. I have used these agents, singly and in combination, with and without zinc and magnesium supplements, for years because of such reports. I have yet to find a definite responder, although it may have been possible that the responses were so subtle that they were not noticed. GLA has been reported to have effects on the noradrenergic autoreceptor and may have decreased palpitations in this manner. Its most predictable response is improving brittle fingernails.

Zinc has been suggested to act as an antioxidant by binding to specific substances that would be pro-oxidants. It must be given in supraphysiologic doses to have this effect. It may act by increasing the body's zinc-metallothionene pool. Cytokines appear to decrease zinc concentrations. Zinc and other essential nutrients are important for thymic function and cell-mediated immunity.[40]

Treating inhalant allergies and food sensitivities in the usual manner, i.e., by antihistamine, corticosteroid and cromolyn nasal sprays, and avoidance of provocative substances, can be beneficial for fatigue and other CFS symptoms. I have not been impressed with the efficacy of hyposensitization in my patients who have tried it. Surgery to improve sinus drainage is sometimes very helpful. The role of diet in CFS is controversial. I suggest that my patients be on a low tyramine diet, and avoid simple sugars, caffeine, alcohol, and nicotine. Some also do well by eliminating red meat, although I have two patients who feel greatly energized whenever they eat it. The enteric nervous system releases a large number of transmitter substances after eating which have the capacity to alter limbic function. If transmitter secretion or limbic receptors are dysregulated, patients could have unusual sensations associated with eating.

Exercise has an immunologic function.[41] Marathon runners frequently get flu-like illnesses after competing, and Olympic athletes get a wide variety of unusual infections. Exercise causes cytokine release, although the function of this process is obscure. It is probably part of the stress response. Slowly graduated exercise may desensitize limbic cytokine receptors. General fitness may play a role as well, since we have noticed that patients who were very active athletically prior to their illness tended to have less severe symptoms than those who were sedentary. We have measured levels of IL-1, cortisol, growth hormone, and other neuroendocrine parameters in CFS patients before and after exercise.[42]

Leuprolide acetate (Lupron) may have an immunomodulatory

role. John Mathias, working at the University of Texas in Galveston, has been using it in various autoimmune disorders with some success.[43] My CFS patients on Lupron for IBS or endometriosis do not report any general symptomatic improvement.

The results of a peptide T trial in AIDS patients has recently been reported.[44] There was no significant change in immune parameters, but there was an improvement in neuropsychiatric symptoms. Although peptide T was designed to block the action of gp120 at the CD4 receptor,[45] which is also the VIP receptor, perhaps its mechanism of action is not immunologic but neuromodulatory. Peptide T may act in AIDS (and CFS) by being a VIP agonist. VIP may stimulate the secretion of IL-1[46] and is stored in nerve fibers with nitric oxide synthase in the outer, adventitial layers of large cerebral blood vessels.[47] The drug is quite safe. It was used because peptide T and VIP can prevent gp120-induced neuronal cell death in vitro. gp120 is the HIV surface molecule that binds to the CD4 receptor and has some sequence homology to VIP. It has been suggested that peptide T may have neurocognitive effects independent of its antiviral activity. A patient with CFS has had a good result using peptide T. We are planning a peptide T trial in CFS.

Amantadine may have some utility in CFS. It is a mild dopamine agonist used in Parkinson's disease, and, as such, may stimulate opioids. It has activity against influenza A, and has been reported to decrease fatigue in patients with multiple sclerosis. Some CFS patients who take amantadine chronically report that they have fewer flu-like illnesses. The *adamantan* compounds, of which amantadine is one, have been investigated for psychotropic and immunomodulatory properties. One such agent is *Kemantan,* developed in Moscow. It has shown great efficacy when used in the Russian equivalent of CFS patients,[48] but cannot be used in the United States. We are conducting in vitro studies of Kemantan on NK function.

Numerous agents which block the synthesis of, or receptors for, cytokines are being developed, although none, excepting perhaps cyclosporin, are clinically available. Substances which increase synthesis of central cytokines, or block the action of their inhibitors, have not been described.

It may be possible to treat CFS by modulating neuroendocrine parameters. Agents to consider would be corticosteroids, ACTH, thyroid hormone, TRH, serotonin agonists, DDAVP to stimulate CRH secretion, and agents to augment growth hormone secretion. These substances have complex interrelationships and many have not been well studied in fatigue states or stress. My experience with them in CFS treatment has generally not been rewarding. Recent attention has been drawn to the possibility of hyposecretion of CRH in CFS causing a central hypocortisolemia and the assertion that CFS is a hormonal disorder.

In an article entitled "Evidence for impaired activation of the hypothalamic-pituitary-adrenal axis in patients with chronic fatigue syndrome," Demitrack et al.[49] studied the functional integrity of various components of the HPA axis in patients who met CDC criteria for CFS. A mild glucocorticoid deficiency was found. The most robust result was 24-hour urinary free cortisol secretion, which was almost half that of normals. ACTH response to CRH was blunted, and there was a reduced maximal adrenal response to ACTH, perhaps demonstrating a degree of adrenal atrophy due to chronic understimulation. Basal plasma evening ACTH levels were elevated, which rules out pituitary insufficiency, but CSF CRH levels were normal.

These researchers suggest that many of the symptoms of CFS, including "debilitating fatigue, an abrupt onset precipitated by a stress or feverishness, arthralgias, myalgias, adenopathy, post-exertional fatigue, exacerbation of allergic responses, and disturbances in mood and sleep are all characteristic of glucocorticoid insufficiency." CRH levels are postulated by these investigators to be low in all neurasthenic states, including Cushing syndrome, hypothyroidism, and seasonal affective disorder. They note that aside from its effects on ACTH secretion, CRH is involved in activation of the sympathetic nervous system, hypervigilance, and increased motor activity. It is suggested that the immune abnormalities seen in CFS are epiphenomena due to impaired glucocorticoid mediation of the immune response. They note that viral infections can alter neurotransmitter and neuroendocrine release, although they seem to favor a post-viral syndrome, rather than an ongoing viral infection, as the cause of such symptoms. The group did not appear to take into account the role of central CRH in mediating central IL-1 beta immunosuppression.

In many respects this theory makes sense. It is a unifying hypothesis, one of the few we have in CFS, and central hypocortisolemia may play a role in post-traumatic stress disorder, which I have postulated to have a role in some cases of CFS, particularly in victims of child abuse. It would involve dysfunction of the hippocampal inhibitory regulation of cortisol secretion, and perhaps that of the amygdala, as well, which secretes CRH in stress situations.[50] The amygdala may be unique among limbic structures in that it has direct neural connections with the neocortical, hypothalamic, and brain stem preganglionic autonomic areas. Altered sensitivity of hippocampal glucocorticoid receptors may also play a role. Antidepressants may act directly at the genomic level to influence glucocorticoid receptor mRNA levels.[51] Chronic stress of one particular type (as opposed to several types) seems to cause an adaptation in the sensitivity of HPA activation in the form of a heightened negative feedback, perhaps to prevent harmful sequelae of chronically elevated glucocorticoid levels. In young rats, a chronic exposure to handling results in an elevated glucocorticoid receptor concentration in the brain which might produce hypocortisolemia and decreased levels of CRH. It has been suggested that due to the effect of cortisol's activating limbic structures, those with hypocortisolemia may produce trait characteristics of passive avoidance behavior as a means of coping. Injection of CRH into the ventricles is anxiogenic.[52]

In the Demitrack study lymphocyte glucocorticoid receptors were not measured. They are increased in post-traumatic stress disorder (PTSD).[53] Dexamethasone suppression was not done. One might expect a hyperresponsivity to this test if cortisol is low and receptors are high. CRH lymphocyte receptors could also be measured. CRH is lowered in brains of patients with Alzheimer's disease, Parkinson's disease, and progressive supranuclear palsy, but not Huntington's disease.[54] Cortical CRH receptors are elevated in the first three of these disorders.

There are serious problems with the postulate that CRH deficiency is the cause of CFS. I attempted to treat numerous patients with evidence of secondary adrenal insufficiency several years ago by replacing their endogenous corticosteroids with prednisone. No patient got more than a replacement dose, and no patient felt better.

Attempts to treat these patients with ACTH have met with limited success. One wonders whether improvement might not be due in some cases to supraphysiologic levels of cortisol. CRH stimulates TRH secretion, and it is possible that some CFS patients have mild tertiary hypothyroidism on the basis of CRH hyposecretion, particularly those with mild hypothyroid indices who do not have increased TSH levels. TRH testing might show a blunted response in such patients.

The CRH measurements in the Demitrack experiment were done by lumbar puncture. Higher values are obtained by cisternal puncture, indicating a rostro-caudal gradient. Differences between the CFS patients and the control group could have been missed because a lumbar puncture was performed rather than a cisternal puncture. Local hyposecretion of CRH could have been more readily detected in this manner. CRH secretion varies over time, and both hypothalamic and extra-hypothalamic CRH are measured by a single lumbar puncture. Placement of a lumbar subarachnoid catheter allows for serial CRH measurement.[55]

Interestingly, CRH is greatly elevated in pregnancy, particularly during the last trimester. The CRH is mostly bound and produced by the placenta, but one wonders whether it produces immunosuppression and could be related to the symptomatic improvement that most pregnant CFS patients experience.

Use of alpha-helical CRH, a CRH antagonist, has not been reported in humans to my knowledge. It may suppress some of the anxiogenic effects of CRH, but not in the manner of benzodiazepines. It apparently must be given i.c.v. since CRH, a 41-amino acid peptide, does not pass the blood-brain barrier well. This fact could limit the use of alpha-helical CRH in humans.

Patients with CFS have been described as being hypervigilant, demonstrating somatosensory amplification, and having overly active sympathetic nervous systems. They are commonly afflicted with panic attacks. All of these symptoms are incompatible with CFS being caused by CRH deficiency. The marked degree of cognitive impairment seen in many patients would also be inconsistent with the rather mild degree of CRH deficiency implied by the Demitrack experiment. I would favor an etiologic hypothesis of primary limbic (e.g., amygdalar and hippocampal) dysfunction causing minor CRH abnormalities, although there may be a subset of CFS patients who would respond to strategies to enhance CRH secretion or to increase adrenal corticosteroids. I have tried fenfluramine and DDAVP, but the combination does not appear to be effective.

If patients have secondary adrenal insufficiency, that should be reflected in inadequate cortisol secretion after exercise and perhaps impaired catecholamine secretion as well. We are in the process of assessing these variables. Preliminary results suggest that most CFS patients do not increase their cortisol as expected after maximal exercise. Exercise testing may be a better functional way than ACTH testing to assess secondary adrenal insufficiency.

The concept of central hypocortisolemia is inconsistent with CFS being an immune activation state of cytokine excess, since all cytokines tested stimulate cortisol secretion. IL-1 stimulates CRH secretion, and CRH upregulates IL-1 receptors. The only way that I can resolve this paradox is to hypothesize that there are increased amounts of cytokine antagonists in the brain that prevent stimulation of CRH secretion, or that there is some basic cellular or eicosanoid deficit that prevents its secretion in response to cytokines. A CNS CRH deficiency could cause a decrease of immunosuppression, or immune activation, in the periphery. A cellular metabolic defect inhibiting central CRH secretion could occur from heredity, environmental factors, infectious agents, or various combinations of all three. The modulation of sympathetic nervous system tone by CRH leads us to consideration of the role of the autonomic nervous system (ANS) and of neurotransmission in general in CFS. It is common for CFS patients to have symptoms such as low blood pressure and night sweats. Wessely et al. found that patients with low blood pressure felt tired all the time, even when adjustment was made for psychiatric illness.[56]

The role of the ANS in human pathophysiology is expanding. I have alluded to cortical control of cardiovascular responsiveness, but there is a cerebellar component as well. State changes, such as sleep and wakefulness, modulate baroreceptor tone, probably by serotoninergic mechanisms. The raphe nuclei are involved in migraine headache patients, in whom there is an impairment of sympathetic outflow to the pupil on the affected side.[57] Migraines are probably more common in CFS. Thermoreceptive neurons in the preoptic area have been shown to be sensitive to behavioral changes or baroreceptor mechanisms. In multiple system atrophy (MSA), glutamic acid decarboxylase (GAD), a marker for GABA, is decreased, especially in the dentate nucleus. GABA agonists, available in other countries, may therefore be useful.[58] A new drug, DL-dops, may increase plasma norepinephrine levels, and somatostatin, which has been occasionally helpful in CFS treatment, ameliorates post-prandial hypotension. These may be employed in MSA. There are infectious causes of autonomic nerve damage, best known in Chagas' disease, but increasingly recognized in AIDS, in which a significant decline in autonomic function is found. Patients with IBS have been noted to have generalized or patchy anhidrosis, evidence of sympathetic denervation. This finding accords well with the work of Mathias, who has found GnRH receptors in sympathetic ganglia which may be one site of action for Lupron in IBS.[59] We have previously discussed the function of the ANS in immunomodulation.

Postural hypotension is a hallmark of autonomic failure, and it appears to be related not to cardiac contractility, but to failure of peripheral arterial vasoconstriction, which is overactive in the extremities of CFS patients (Raynaud's disorder) but may be underactive, or dysregulated, elsewhere. I have discussed this issue in the section on fibromyalgia. Sleep apnea has been noted in MSA patients and may be related to the incidence of this disorder in the CFS population.

The CNS mechanisms regulating functional autonomic states have recently been reviewed, mainly concentrating on the cardiovascular system, urinary bladder, and several organs.[60,61] Descending pathways to the pontine parabrachial nuclei mediate patterns of cardiac and respiratory rhythms through GABAergic mechanisms. The parabrachial nuclei project to rostroventrolateral medulla (RVLM). The posterior vermis of the cerebellum, from which some of these fibers come, is essential for acquisition of classically conditioned bradycardias. Baroreceptors and chemoreceptors connect directly with the nucleus tractus solitarius (NTS). The NTS receives a powerful input from limbic and paralimbic areas, mediated by GABAergic neurons. There is evidence that GABAergic neurotransmission is impaired in

CFS (e.g., panic attacks), and the NTS may be dysregulated in a similar fashion. IL-1 receptors are also found in the parabrachial nuclei and the NTS.

Claims have been made that RVLM neurons are responsible for sympathetic tone since they project to sympathetic preganglionic neurons in the thoracic spinal cord. There are "pacemaker" neurons in the RVLM that increase their discharge after application of beta receptor agonists, and beta-blockers may act centrally at this location. The emerging picture is that regulation of the autonomic nervous system is not a "mass response" but is highly differentiated and an example of parallel processing. Various pathways contain specific transmitter substances including amines, peptides, and amino acids, and mediate specific functions via particular populations of preganglionic neurons of the ANS. I have discussed this previously in relation to BAT thermogenesis.

A technique to establish which CFS patients with ANS dysfunction have MSA and which have peripheral autonomic failure (PAF) would be measurement of ACTH and plasma adrenaline after cholinergic challenge, as with arecoline. Acetylcholine also stimulates CRH and GHRH secretion. Patients with both MSA and PAF will fail to increase ACTH levels, but only those with MSA increase plasma adrenaline. My preliminary results would suggest CFS patients fit more into the MSA category which could be caused by central hyposecretion of CRH, a substance which circulates throughout the entire neuraxis.

Drug therapy of orthostatic hypotension is limited to mineralocorticoids and NSAIDs. Inhaled ergotamine is also effective, but chronic use may be a problem because of possible ergotism.

SOMATIZATION DISORDER

From a brief review of the ANS let us turn to somatization disorder, a category into which many CFS patients could fit. The early 1990s must represent the apogee of psychologizing illness much akin to the psychoanalyzing of it during my medical training. When I attempted to introduce the notion of behavior modification in a conference dealing with a man who had a post-traumatic crane phobia after an industrial accident and who had been through four years of psychoanalysis, I was told "people aren't rats," and that was the end of that.

Nowadays, in a more scientifically advanced medical environment, people *are* like rats at times. The pain clinic environment popularized by Fordyce works by not reinforcing pain behavior. It can reduce pain perception in many cases of chronic pain by operant conditioning. More sophisticated programs add cognitive-behavioral therapy, which can also be done on an outpatient basis. The same paradigms can apply to the CFS patient as to the chronic pain patient. In a recent work,[62] it is suggested that there are three main mechanisms which act in hypochondriacal states to increase anxiety, as well as to enhance preoccupation with illness and the misinterpretation of bodily variations that characterize unexplained somatic concerns:

1. Increased physiologic arousal, leading to increased occurrence of autonomically mediated sensations;
2. Selective attention (that which has previously been termed somatosensory amplification); and
3. Avoidant behaviors based on perceptions of such symptoms which would constitute illness behavior.

Therapy in a cognitive-behavioral paradigm is aimed at decreasing avoidant behaviors no matter what their cause. These symptoms could also be a result of limbic/prefrontal encephalopathy, however, as previously discussed.

Patients with CFS are often grouped into the category of "functional" disorders, a pejorative term to denote disorders which do not have an ascertainable organic etiology. "Functional" perpetuates the organic/psychological dichotomy, and many CFS patients feel stigmatized by this term, as well as by physicians who turn away from them after it is used.

"Somatization" should be slightly better, but may in fact be worse, because it is interpreted by most physicians to mean the conversion of emotional problems into physical ones, or, at best, the "misattribution" of bodily symptoms as if they were due to "organic" disease. The symptoms are "unaccounted for by pathological findings" (Lipowski).[63]

It used to be thought that somatizers were "alexithymics," people who were incapable of feeling or expressing emotions. Other somatizers are said to have "masked depression," and that their symptoms are expressions of psychological illness. Somatizers, however, have high lifetime expression of anxiety and depression and their symptoms are now thought to be common expressions of distress.[64] "Reattributing" patients' symptoms to genuine expressions of distress is helpful, particularly if a physiologic explanation, such as autonomic overactivity, is invoked. Some experts seem to invoke the cognitive theory of emotion propounded by Schachter and Singer[65] to explain that somatizers misinterpret visceral information to the brain.

Somatization is thought to be common, although only a small minority of CFS patients meet DSM-III-R criteria for the diagnosis. *Attributional style* is a current buzz phrase in cognitive psychology as applied to the somatizer. Focusing on somatic issues by a patient is said to prevent psychological understanding and obscures the need for personal change. The stigma of mental illness may also be avoided, and by somatizing, a patient may lessen the responsibility for whatever life predicament he or she may be in.

Cultural factors are thought to play a large role in somatization and may facilitate entering the medical model. It is thought by many that CFS is like the neurasthenia of the nineteenth century and that it will disappear once it is recognized as a primary psychiatric disorder.[66,67] The prominence of infectious disease and environmental toxicity issues in the late twentieth century are thought to account for the unconscious choice to convert emotional conflicts into symptoms of CFS.

Inability to disclose traumatic childhood events may produce adverse health outcomes by increasing psychological "work," which may manifest itself as increased autonomic activity. This concept sounds suspiciously like repressed id impulses in the psychoanalytic "hydraulic" theory of emotions, and may be better explained by a neurologic process.

International Classification of Disease-10 (ICD-10) is a little better than DSM-III-R in categorizing somatoform disorders. The draft of ICD-10 has a category for "psychogenic autonomic dysfunction" as well as "Neurasthenia (fatigue syndrome)."[68] In general, the subcategories of somatoform disorders in both manuals lack specific defining characteristics to distinguish one from another. I do not wish to enter the thicket of nosology in this book. I would rather emphasize what I consider to be the underlying biologic mechanisms, a focus strangely ignored by almost all studying the subject.

It is difficult to get some CFS patients to see that there might be psychiatric aspects to their symptoms, much less to treat their illness as a primary psychiatric disorder. Furthermore, health insurance often will not pay for psychiatric care, and disability will reimburse less, or not at all, for a "nervous and mental disorder."

Still, one should look for somatic complaints accompanying life changes, parental illness and learning of the sick role, the impact of illnesses in childhood, and normal medical interventions for somatic complaints. It is thought that somatizing patients have a diathesis to express depression and anxiety as changes in somatic and motor function exclusively, rather than alterations as well in mood and thought content and social function and behavior.

Many patients with CFS hyperventilate (about 15 percent in our series). The reasons why they should do so have not really been addressed to my satisfaction, but the symptoms of hyperventilation have been well described by Bass and Gardner,[69] and possible mechanisms of symptom production are proposed, which are mainly consequences of respiratory alkalosis. Chest pain, palpitations, dizziness, syncope, unilateral somatic symptoms, air hunger, dry mouth, flatulence, belching, abdominal distension, esophageal spasm, poor concentration, forgetfulness, unusual psychosensory experiences, weakness, and listlessness are described. We are, however, somewhat able to differentiate by clinical criteria those who hyperventilate from those who do not. Patients who have fibromyalgia tender points are more likely to hyperventilate. Clues are a history of air hunger or atypical chest pain. The three-minute hyperventilation provocation test is useful.[70] Behavioral treatments for hyperventilation are not successful very often. Treating CFS patients who hyperventilate with medications for anxiety such as tricyclic antidepressants, fluoxetine, buspirone, beta blockers, and

MAOIs, while quite helpful, is no more helpful than in treating the non-hyperventilating CFS patients. Although my preference for the mechanism of hyperventilation involves amygdalar dysfunction in a pathway to the pneumotaxic center in the pons,[71] Dr. Paul Cheney believes it is a response to benign intracranial hypertension caused by virally induced cell damage. A popular etiology is the dysregulation of medullary chemoreceptors. Hyperventilation at the onset of exercise, seen in some CFS patients, may be due to a decreased endorphinergic suppression of ventilation.

We do not find cognitive-behavioral therapy (CBT) as useful in the sense of *reattribution* as we do in *reframing*, enabling patients to live within the confines of their disabilities and still being able to be as productive as possible. The two main complaints, fatigue and cognitive dysfunction, are both often quite severe and are difficult to reattribute, although the less severe symptoms of autonomic hyperactivity respond better to such interventions. CBT in CFS aims at increasing activity, working on the assumption that since activity worsened symptoms during the acute viral phase of the illness, a CFS patient gets the mistaken belief that activity will worsen his condition during later stages of the illness, refrains from activity, becomes deconditioned, and feels worse when he exerts himself because he: (a) expects to; (b) is out of shape; and (c) has somatosensory amplification. The patient is asked to continue exercising even though symptoms may increase. Exercise must be slowly graduated. A gradual return to normal activities is also encouraged.

I have no problem with most of these recommendations, adopted from Simon Wessely et al., except that I do not insist that a patient continue exercising when his exercise has caused him to relapse. I have many patients who cannot tolerate this program, particularly if they relapse in the middle of it for no apparent reason.

I believe that a thorough psychosocial history should be taken from the CFS patient, and that one should be empathic with past distressing experiences, allowing the patient to "abreact." It is difficult for the general medical physician to find the time for this sort of relationship when symptoms and medications must be reviewed and charted and a physical must be done. Furthermore, many of my patients are referred to me by psychotherapists who have already tried this approach and have found it ineffective.

The reattribution that I do is to explain limbic physiology to the patient. I tell him in appropriate terms that I believe his symptoms are caused by a dysfunction of heteromodal and limbic structures and the problem is interactive and possibly multicausal. To the extent that there are impaired cognitions (which would include anticipatory anxiety as well as somatosensory amplification), I invoke dysfunction in the heteromodal and paralimbic areas, which can directly affect limbic centers as well as the brain stem and spinal cord. Heteromodal and paralimbic dysregulation would be amenable to CBT. Successful psychotherapy must produce neurochemical changes as well as attitudinal ones. Alterations in caudate metabolic rate in patients with obsessive-compulsive disorder have been demonstrated in PET scans of patients treated either with fluoxetine or CBT.[72] Certain symptoms may respond better to one type of therapy or the other. If there is an indication of PTSD from child abuse or other trauma that is not being discussed, "uncovering" therapy would be appropriate. Although exploration of "secondary gain" in CFS might seem appropriate to some, I do not find it useful. I have discussed graduated exercise previously. I find pain clinics more effective for pain than for fatigue. Relaxation techniques and biofeedback are of some limited value in disorders of autonomic hyperactivity.

Since I do not know of non-CBT ways to alter heteromodal association area activity, except perhaps by the use of nootropics, my paradigm for CFS treatment otherwise is organic. I have already discussed antiviral and immunomodulatory therapies. I would like to reemphasize that in a double-blind trial, Ampligen helped CFS symptoms without regard to how depressed a patient was or when in his lifetime he became depressed. This result, in and of itself, should cause many to re-examine their notions of the pathogenesis of CFS.

NEUROPHARMACOLOGY OF CFS

The neuropharmacological approach to CFS is, in many ways, similar to the treatment of panic disorder, except that CFS patients respond to lower doses of medication, have more adverse drug reactions, and do not respond as well to this strategy as do patients with "pure" panic disorder. Recall that panic disorder patients sensitive to lactate challenge showed increased activity in the parahippocampal gyrus on PET scans,[73] but that this finding has been related to masseter and temporalis contraction as a result of bruxism.[74]

The mainstays of treatment are benzodiazepines, tricyclic antidepressants, monoamine oxidase inhibitors (MAOIs), fluoxetine and sertraline. All these agents are effective in panic disorder and generalized anxiety disorder. None of the benzodiazepines (except for alprazolam) are effective in treating depression. Panic disorder with accompanying depression will not respond as well unless the depression is treated also. Angiotensin converting enzyme inhibitors such as captopril, when used as antidepressants or enkephalinase inhibitors for pain, have weak effects. Sodium valproate (Depakote) may also be useful in panic disorder and PTSD.[75]

I have had the experience on numerous occasions of successfully treating CFS depression and anxiety, which may often be viewed as comorbid disorders, with pharmacologic agents only to have the fatigue, cognitive dysfunction, pain, and other symptoms persist. It is somewhat unusual to have all CFS symptoms eliminated with one of these medications. Judging by their efficacy in panic disorder, the MAOIs should be the best medication to treat CFS patients.[76] They are also good drugs to use in "atypical" depressions, which are perhaps those with low CRH levels. I have tried phenelzine (Nardil) and tranylcypromine (Parnate) in hundreds of CFS patients, and selegiline (Eldepryl) in scores. I have only a handful of patients on these medications chronically. This response suggests to me that although CFS and panic disorder/depression may seem to be different names for the same disorder, that appearance may conflict with reality. Somatization disorder is also reported to preferentially respond to MAOIs.[77] Antidepressants of various sorts interfere with CRH activity in the region of the locus ceruleus, either by blocking its effect (phenelzine) or attenuating its release (desipramine). These mechanisms do not explain the response to antidepressants in low CRH states. MAOIs increase dopamine levels, while heterocyclics do not. This differential effect may suggest that atypical depression involves a dopamine deficiency in the limbic striatum, namely in the mesoprefrontal and mesocingulate pathways. This deficiency may be due to decreased catecholamine and serotonin stimulation at the mu receptor by beta endorphin.[78] Peripheral immune activation, often found in CFS, could thus be related to low central beta-endorphin activity at certain sites. I have used MAOIs successfully in patients with deafferentation syndrome, a disorder influenced in part by limbic mechanisms. Atypical depression responds much better to MAOIs than to tricyclics.[79] The "Columbia Criteria" for probable or definite atypical depression are:

a. mood reactivity when depressed
b. two (one for probable) associated features:
   hyperphagia, hypersomnia, leaden paralysis, and pathologic sensitivity to interpersonal rejection as a trait throughout adulthood.[80]

Many CFS patients could be diagnosed as having atypical depression, although mood reactivity when depressed is not a prominent feature of most CFS patients I have seen, nor is hyperphagia or rejection sensitivity.

Buspirone, an agent effective in anxiety, depression, addictive disorders, and attention deficit, is not too useful in CFS. It is not an effective treatment for panic disorder and most authorities consider it to be less effective than alternative therapies. Its main advantages in CFS are in augmenting the effect of fluoxetine or tricyclics. It cannot be used with MAOIs or bupropion, and may have its best effect in those who have never taken benzodiazepines.

I have had poor results using bupropion (Wellbutrin) in CFS patients with prominent anxiety symptoms, but it is sometimes effective when no other drug is. Bupropion is most useful in those with fatigue as the main complaint, although sometimes all symptoms will resolve, including pain.

The idea that some CFS patients have a form of post-traumatic stress disorder (PTSD) is an attractive one, since a history of child abuse is fairly common, and so is high life stress prior to onset of illness. Post et al.[81] popularized the notion of kindling as a biological model for progressively developing symptoms in psychiatric disorders, and it is an attractive hypothesis to explain why CFS symptoms are so sensitive to minor stressors which could have previously been well tolerated. Kindling is a concept which began in epilepsy research. Repetitive stimulation below the threshold to induce a seizure would eventually cause one. Spontaneous seizures could then be the result of chronic kindling. It was suggested that repetitive stress-induced limbic system neurobiologic alterations could progressively affect function in a similar manner.

In an important paper in which he postulates that "both sensitization to stressors and episode sensitization occur and become encoded at the level of gene expression, Post writes:

> The quality of the stressor may similarly affect specific neural systems based not only on the type and location of short-term biochemical changes but also on the type, location, mixture, and interaction of oncogenes and transcription factors, with differential consequences for subsequent coding of long-term protein and peptide changes. Psychosocial stresses involving losses and threats of losses in a social context may have very different cognitive, behavioral, and neurobiological consequences from stresses involving the threat of bodily injury, which may be more pertinent to the induction of syndromes such as posttraumatic stress disorder (PTSD).[82]

PTSD apparently is associated with decreased CRH levels and also with dysfunction of the sympathetic nervous system. Lithium, carbamazepine (Tegretol), and sodium valproate (Depakote) are all effective treatments for PTSD, reducing kindling and autonomic arousal by stimulating GABAergic neurons. Carbamazepine and valproate are increasingly used for bipolar disorders, schizoaffective disorder, and treatment-resistant depression. Valproate is useful in anxiety and panic disorder, as well as in migraine headaches.

PTSD may be characterized by loss of inhibitory cortical (heteromodal and paralimbic) control over limbic structures involved in arousal and alarm, producing activation of the sympathetic nervous system and flashbacks which might continue limbic kindling, a state which manifests an increase in benzodiazepine receptors. Sympathetic overactivity, however, would not be predicted by a low CRH state, a problem with this model.

I have found lithium to be of almost no use in CFS, and have tried it many times, usually as antidepressant augmentation. It has no intrinsic value in CFS aside from its usual indications. Carbamazepine is similarly unhelpful, and the only patients of mine who are still taking it are those with temporolimbic epilepsy. Few of my patients take valproate, but it is effective for an occasional patient who has panic disorder and cannot tolerate, or does not respond to, other agents. It has no effect on fatigue, cognitive dysfunction, pain, or flu-like symptoms, and little effect on other symptoms.

Although the incidence of hypothyroidism, perhaps on a central basis, appears to be increased in CFS patients, antidepressant augmentation with thyroid hormone, either T_4 or T_3, has not proven to be a useful strategy, and I rarely even try it any longer. It is possible that some CFS patients have hyposecretion of TRH. This peptide stimulates CRH secretion and sympathetic nervous system activity, effects which are independent of each other, since the stimulation of CRH can be antagonized by specific agents but the augmentation of the SNS persists.[83] A cyclization metabolic product of the tripeptide TRH, His-Pro-DKP, antagonizes ethanol narcosis,[84] and a deficiency of TRH might explain the ethanol hypersensitivity manifested by most CFS patients. TRH is also co-localized with serotonin in raphe nuclei, and this is certainly reason to suspect CFS is a serotonin deficiency state, although measurements of CSF 5-HIAA have been done in FM patients in whom they are low.[85] 5-HIAA levels have been reported as being normal in CFS patients.[86] The physiologic effects of TRH have been discussed previously. The transmitter regulation of TRH secretion is not well understood, despite two decades of research. TRH secretion appears to be inhibited by GABA and dopamine. Results with serotonin have been contradictory, and trials with numerous neuropeptides have been unproductive. Currently available agents to block dopamine and GABA are not effective in CFS. TRH treatment of depression has not been successful. A major regulator of TRH secretion could be IL-1 beta.

Added to the relative lack of success of traditional panic disorder treatments (especially benzodiazepines) to eliminate most CFS symptoms, a medication that is acutely effective for panic is the alpha-2 agonist clonidine. This agent, which appears to work by decreasing the firing of the locus ceruleus, is not at all helpful for CFS symptoms, except night sweats. A hypothesis which tries to reconcile paradigms of panic disorder being either a biologic or a behavioral disorder considers the role of the locus ceruleus in an integrative manner. In the article, "A Neuroanatomical Hypothesis for Panic Disorder," Gorman et al. in 1989[87] relate the acute panic attack to the brain stem, especially the locus ceruleus, but also the medullary chemoreceptors and the serotoninergic dorsal raphe. The brain stem nuclei are thought to be hypersensitive, causing a cascade of neural events responsible for panic. These structures relate to provocation of panic attacks in susceptible patients by lactate, carbon dioxide, isoproterenol, and yohimbine. Such experiments have not been performed in CFS patients. Vertigo in panic disorder patients could be caused by pontine discharges to the cerebellar centers that control vestibular function. CFS vertigo, however, responds inconstantly to panic disorder medication. Phenelzine seems the most effective. An attractive aspect of this hypothesis is that these putative brain stem loci for panic can be readily stimulated by descending pathways originating in higher cortical centers. Results of direct stimulation and ablation of the locus ceruleus in animal models have been contradictory as far as the etiology of panic disorder is concerned. Gorman's group now thinks that panic disorder is a type of somatosensory amplification produced by attitudinal and/or brain stem dysfunction.[88]

It is suggested that locus ceruleus inhibition of hippocampal activity produces anxiety. Benzodiazepines may reduce generalized anxiety but not sodium lactate induced panic. Since benzodiazepine receptors are dense in limbic structures, it may be that these anxiolytics act there but not in the brain stem. There are well-known pathways from the limbic system to the locus ceruleus. Gorman et al. suggest that "repeated stimulation of limbic neurons by brain stem discharge lowers the threshold to excitatory postsynaptic stimulation in the limbic lobe until 'subpanic' stimulation is capable of maintaining the 'kindled' anticipatory anxiety. Thus, even without the further occurrence of panic, the limbic area continues to have a reduced threshold for response to various stressors." It may be that the hyperventilation that accompanies panic attacks causes reduced cerebral blood flow in the limbic system and is thereby responsible for the symptoms of hyperventilation syndrome. In our CFS SPECT scan population, the patients who chronically hyperventilated (as determined by end-tidal pCO_2) could be symptomatically distinguished from those who did not only by the presence of fibromyalgia tender points. Addition of agents which markedly increase cerebral blood flow, such as calcium channel blockers (except for nimodipine) and acetazolamide, do not often reduce such symptoms. Patients with anxiety disorders, however, have normal, or increased, cerebral blood flow.[89] Acetazolamide lowers brain pH but causes hyperventilation.

A review of the literature on the role of hypocapnia in agoraphobia, generalized anxiety disorder, and panic disorder yields contradictory results in the pathogenesis of these disorders. It seems that hyperventilation in and of itself may produce abnormal cognitive, affective, and somatic sensations, depending on the way the experience is perceived by the patient. This tendency, variously termed "anxiety sensitivity," "catastrophic interpretation" or "somatosensory amplification," has been discussed previously. It is thought by some that the various agents used to provoke panic, e.g., lactate, caffeine, yohimbine, isoproterenol, 5% CO_2, naloxone, bicarbonate, etc., have little in common. Others relate all of their effects to the relationship between CO_2 and norepinephrine at the level of the locus ceruleus. Some proponents of the biological model suggest that patients with panic attacks may chronically hyperventilate in an attempt to maintain a low CO_2 level to avoid triggering supposed hypersensitive central noradrenergic CO_2 receptors. Hyperventilation during panic attacks would thus be an unsuccessful way of reducing large adrenergic discharges. Acetazolamide, which increases local CO_2 tension by inhibiting carbonic anhydrase, does not cause anxiety in CFS patients, but does not often seem to decrease it, either.

It is also difficult to reconcile the hyperventilation hypothesis with low CRH levels and decreased activity of the sympathetic nervous system, but it may be true that anticipatory anxiety, if a limbic phenomenon, could reach levels high enough to trigger locus ceruleus discharge by descending mechanisms. Antipanic medications as well as cognitive-behavioral interventions could alter the threshold for such limbic activation.

A view which I favor is that panic attacks are primarily a limbic, and not a brain stem, phenomenon, since alprazolam may block even lactate-induced panic. In some studies the CFS panic disorder, particularly in those patients with no premorbid mood disorders, seems to be somewhat different. The anticipatory anxiety seems to be much more autonomous, as if it were being generated by a neurotransmitter disorder, as one might see in a post-viral syndrome. Once again, most CFS symptoms do not usually resolve when panic attacks and anxiety are reduced or even eliminated. This clinical observation supports the hypothesis that a limbic encephalopathy is involved with most cases of CFS, and that one aspect of this process would be panic disorder.

It is hypothesized that the prefrontal cortex generates agoraphobia by stimulus generalization as a result of random panic attacks. I prefer to interpret agoraphobia as being a dysfunction of heteromodal and paralimbic input to limbic structures and not to restrict agoraphobia to the prefrontal cortex. However, a "panic disorder circuit" has been proposed from the medullary reticular area to the locus ceruleus, through the dorsal ascending bundle to the limbic lobe and prefrontal cortex and back to the nucleus reticularis gigantocellularis, which gives primary stimulatory input to the locus ceruleus. My view would involve more cortical structures. This circuit would include structures found to be hypoperfused in CFS brain SPECT scans, the anterior temporal lobe and the dorsolateral prefrontal cortex.

There is a genetic tendency to develop panic attacks. There may also be a learned tendency to catastrophize from heteromodal/paralimbic information, thereby provoking panic attacks. This neuroanatomical hypothesis makes sense for panic disorder, but not for the multitude of CFS symptoms that would be difficult to fit under the panic disorder aegis. Anti-kindling medications are not particularly effective in CFS, and benzodiazepines rarely affect symptoms other than anxiety, vertigo, or IBS (for which they are very effective).

Calcium channel blockers have anti-anxiety effects,[90,91] but only nimodipine is of much value in CFS. Nifedepine has been used in epilepsy. A possible use for them would be in combination with acetazolamide and magnesium to interfere with excitotoxin release after cell injury, caused by various possible factors, especially viruses. Magnesium itself has been reported to prevent panic attacks in the so-called "neuronal hyperexcitability syndrome" as well as anxiety and somatization. Depression was not affected. Nimodipine has been most tested in an ischemic model designed to stimulate release of excitatory amino acids (EAAs) and is the calcium channel blocker that I have had the best, although limited, results with in CFS. Ischemia has marked effects in the hippocampus, particularly in the CA1 region, and nimodipine attenuates ischemic damage there. It also improves cerebral blood flow and enhances protection by MK-801, a glutamate antagonist. I have discussed the possible role of Peptide T in this paradigm previously. Nimodipine also inhibits cerebral hypermetabolism, seizure, and contraction of cerebral resistance vessels in rats, when endothelin is given intraventricularly. The subsequent reduction in blood flow is thought to be mediated by dihydropyridine sensitive L-channels.[92,93] Nimodipine effectively treated panic disorder in patients who had decreases in basilar artery blood flow as measured by transcranial Doppler of greater than 80%. Responders had normalization in their basilar mean flow velocity and pulsatility index responses to hyperventilation after nimodipine treatment. Non-responders, which are more typical, had only a 50% reduction in basilar flow velocity after hyperventilation. Thus "only a subset of patients with panic disorder and severe hyperventilation-induced ischemia might benefit from nimodipine or other centrally active calcium channel antagonists."[94] Although I have found nicardipine or isradipine effective in treating the vasoregulatory asthenia subset of CFS, nimodipine may be dramatically effective in those with brain SPECT hypoperfusion. Calcium channel blockers are also useful in migraine, seizure disorders, altitude sickness, anxiety, phobias, Tourette's syndrome, and bipolar affective disorder. Toxicity may develop if they are used concomitantly with other anticonvulsants. A few patients have had increased cognition and energy while taking nimodipine and are unable to discontinue it without relapse. Nitric oxide deficiency may account for vasoconstriction as well as deficits in immune regulation[95] (see Figure 2). It could conceivably be replaced by long-acting nitrates, which are metabolized to nitric oxide, or by L-arginine, which is converted equally into nitric oxide and citrulline via nitric oxide synthase.[96]

Protein kinase C (PKC) is also increased by EAA neurotoxicity. I have attempted to inhibit this enzyme with phenobarbital in CFS

FIGURE 2. Nitric oxide goes centre stage

Forget, for 10 minutes or so, about those countless proteins and other complicated molecules, all with horrendous names, that regulate our bodily functions. Consider instead one of the simplest possible substances—nitric oxide. A free radical, difficult to measure because its half life is only a few seconds, nitric oxide is now the focus of worldwide research considerably more intensive than that which went into the early work on DNA and on the structures of hormones and enzymes.

In less than a decade, this elementary gas (not to be confused with the anesthetic nitrous oxide) has been found to have a staggering range of physiological roles, and has grabbed centre stage accordingly. Nitric oxide is the messenger through which the white cells known as macrophages attack and destroy cancer cells and invading bacteria. It is also the substance which, released from endothelium in response to acetylcholine and other vasodilators, makes blood vessels relax. And now researchers at Johns Hopkins University School of Medicine, Baltimore, have discovered that this deceptively slight molecule mediates penile erection too.

There's more. Nitric oxide occurs in the brain, and suspicions are increasing that it is the prime member of an entirely new class of neurotransmitters. Commenting recently in *Nature* (1992;358: 623) on the introduction of a microsensor that responds to vanishingly tiny quantities of nitric oxide inside and on the surfaces of cells, Solomon Snyder pointed out that in the brain the enzyme that synthesises nitric oxide is localised in discrete populations of neurons which are selectively resistant of neurotoxic damage as a result of stroke and Huntingdon's disease. In the peripheral autonomic nervous system, the enzyme occurs also in neurons to the adrenal medulla and posterior pituitary and in those that regulate peristalsis in the intestine. In all of these systems nitric oxide operates as a neurotransmitter, released as a consequence of nerve stimulation.

But a new *class* of neurotransmitters? It was 1914 when Henry Dale began the classical work on acetylcholine for which, in 1936, he shared a Nobel prize with Otto Loewi. Surely nerve transmission has been so thoroughly researched over the intervening decades that, with the quirky exception of nitric oxide, little more remains to be learned?

Apparently not. The next candidate for recognition alongside nitric oxide as an atypical neuronal messenger is another disarmingly simple molecule, carbon monoxide. Although poisonous when inhaled, carbon monoxide is generated in the body by haem oxygenase. And recent work has shown that this enzyme exists in two forms. One occurs in the spleen and other tissues associated with the destruction of red blood cells, but the other is abundant in the brain. There it may well fulfil subtle functions as another hitherto unsuspected agent of nerve transmission.

It's often said that medical students spend unconscionable amounts of time digesting bucketloads of metabolic complexity. Perhaps, at long last, the really essential chemistry is becoming simple?

—Bernard Dixon,
European contributing editor,
Biotechnology

patients with no therapeutic results. Remember that protein kinase C activity was found to be decreased in the lymphocytes of fibromyalgia patients. Activators of PKC enhance synaptic transmission. PKC may be responsible for a prolonged phase of calcium activation. Enzymes that may contribute to EAA activity[97] are calpains I and II; phospholipase A_2, which produces arachidonic acid which may activate PKC; phospholipase C which generates IP_3 which raises cytosolic Ca^{++} by releasing it from internal stores and also raises diacylglycerol, which activates PKC and may enhance glutamate release. Nitric oxide synthase is also released, which should cause arterial dilatation, but also generates free radicals, as do other of these enzymes. The vasoconstriction seen in CFS brain SPECT scans may result from inhibition of constitutive nitric oxide synthase activity. Magnesium depleted or injured cells tolerate EAA toxicity poorly because they may not be able to secrete enough magnesium to inhibit EAA secretion. The major damage by EAAs is caused by opening of calcium channels permitting intra- and extracellular influx to exceed efflux, producing cell damage and possibly death. Besides agents already mentioned, $LiCO_3$ inhibits IP_3, and hydroxychloroquine blocks phospholipase A_2. Neither of these drugs is particularly beneficial in CFS, although CFS may overlap with disorders such as systemic lupus erythematosus or ankylosing spondylitis, in which case hydroxychloroquine would obviously be effective. CFS pathophysiology is more consistent with EAA deficiency than excess.

Other treatment possibilities include (a) substances which increase levels of NADPH, since nitric oxide synthase is NADPH-diaphorase,[98] (b) tetrahydrobiopterin, a cofactor in nitric oxide biosynthesis; and (c) nicotinic and muscarinic cholinergic agonists, since the vasodilatation that occurs during mental work is dependent on acetylcholine stimulation of nitric oxide.[99,100] Flavin adenine dinucleotide and mononucleotide are also nitric oxide synthase cofactors.

Rapidly acting activators of nitric oxide synthase include calcium ionophores, excitatory amino acids, acetylcholine, bradykinin, formylated peptides, leukotrienes, platelet activating factor, and phorbol myristate acetate.[101]

The CNS type of the three forms of nitric oxide synthase is found predominantly in the cerebellum, but not in its Purkinje cells.[102] This fact would implicate the cerebellum in any proposed nitric oxide-dependent CFS neural network.

Since neuronal nitric oxide synthase can be activated by acetylcholine, a rational approach to increasing its activity would be with agonists at the nicotinic and muscarinic cholinergic receptors. Acetylcholine is an important transmitter in the limbic system, and it has been suggested that decreased levels of acetylcholinesterase may be related to somatosensory amplification.[103] Patients with multiple chemical sensitivities have been reported to be very sensitive to both organophosphate insecticides[104] and anticholinergic drugs.[105] These individuals have many features in common with CFS patients.

Nitric oxide may also mediate post-synaptic regulation of pre-synaptic transmitter release. This phenomenon has been studied in the production of long-term potentiation (LTP) by glutamate binding to non-NMDA receptors in the hippocampus. This induction of LTP is dependent on post-synaptic depolarization, calcium influx, and activation of protein and calmodulin kinases. For maintenance of LTP, however, the post-synaptic neuron stimulates the firing pre-synaptic neurons to secrete more transmitter, in this case glutamate. This stimulation may occur by the post-synaptic secretion of nitric oxide which diffuses into the pre-synaptic terminals and stimulates guanylyl cyclase enhancement of transmitter release to maintain LTP[106] (see Figure 3). Multiple firing presynaptic neurons in a neural network could thus cause an integrated increase in transmission via nitric oxide.

Such a mechanism could be impaired if IL-1 beta is a transmitter required to stimulate post-synaptic nitric oxide synthase, as it is in other systems. IL-1 beta inhibitors could then interfere with encoding as well as decrease pre-synaptic transmitter secretion in other situations.

Vasoconstriction may also be a result of cell membrane damage as a result of the glutamate cascade which produces eicosanoids and platelet activating factor.[107] The use of agents to block these compounds has not been particularly helpful in CFS. Inhibiting glutamate secretion by stimulating adenosine receptors with dipyridamole (Persantine) is similarly unhelpful. As previously mentioned,

FIGURE 3

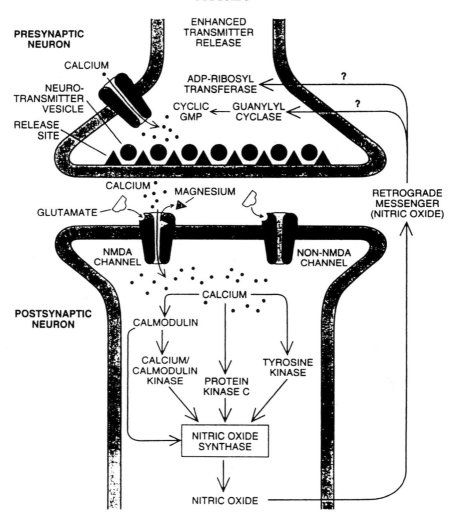

IN LONG-TERM POTENTIATION the postsynaptic membrane is depolarized by the actions of the non-NMDA receptor channels. The depolarization relieves the magnesium blockade of the NMDA channel, allowing calcium to flow through the channel. The calcium triggers calcium-dependent kinases that lead to the induction of LTP. The postsynaptic cell is thought to release a retrograde messenger capable of penetrating the membrane of the presynaptic cell. This messenger, which may be nitric oxide, is believed to act in the presynaptic terminal to enhance transmitter (glutamate) release, perhaps by activating guanylyl cyclase or ADP-ribosyl transferase.

using dextromethorphan to block glutamate receptors has not been useful,[108] even when I have given dextromethorphan to the point of mild toxicity. Increased extracellular fluid acidity reduces NMDA receptor-mediated activity. Acetazolamide (Diamox) can cause a metabolic acidosis. Dihydropyridines given with NMDA antagonists may work better than either agent given alone. When ischemia in experimental animals results in arachidonic acid formation, free radicals are produced. There are numerous strategies to inhibit free radicals. Regional cerebral blood flow in the SPECT scans of some of our CFS patients is low enough that ischemia could occur. The hypothesis that I am developing, however, suggests that EAA levels would be decreased in CFS.

Serotonin pathophysiology in the brain is very complex. What appears obvious is that many patients respond to fluoxetine (Prozac), a serotonin reuptake inhibitor, although fluoxetine may work in CFS by being a $5HT_{1A}$ agonist. Few, however, respond to buspirone, a $5HT_{1A}$ receptor agonist, and none respond to cyproheptadine (Periactin), a serotonin blocker, primarily at the $5HT_2$ receptor. Research that I have done indicates that ritanserin, a $5HT_{1c}/5HT_2$ antagonist, markedly improved some treatment-refractory fibromyalgia patients who had no particular benefit from trazodone (Desyrel), a $5HT_2$ antagonist.[109] Both ritanserin and trazodone increase slow-wave sleep, impaired in CFS by the alpha-EEG abnormality. An interesting aspect of my study was that several patients had a symptomatic rebound after discontinuing ritanserin, an effect which had not been reported previously.[110] Ritanserin by virtue of its ability to increase dopamine release from the nucleus accumbens, may stimulate mesolimbic and mesocortical tracts as well as newly discovered dopamine receptors, D_3-D_5, found in limbic areas.[111] A dopamine deficiency in these regions, unique to CFS/FM, may account for the rebound symptoms patients experienced upon ritanserin discontinuation.[112] Ritanserin is now being tried in drug withdrawal paradigms. No one to my knowledge has treated CFS with sumatriptan, a $5HT_{1D}$ agonist used to treat migraine, or ondansetron, a $5HT_3$ antagonist approved for nausea, which may have anxiolytic and antipsychotic properties. My experience with ondansetron in CFS is that it is not helpful. Ergotamine derivatives, which also block serotonin, have no apparent effect in CFS. All six or seven serotonin receptors are present in the hippocampus. I have treated three CFS patients with migraine headache with IM sumatriptan. All had worsening of symptoms.

The action of mCPP, a potent and reasonably selective agonist at the $5HT_{1c}$ receptor, may shed some light on serotonin effects in CFS. It exacerbates the symptoms of several psychiatric illnesses: anxiety in GAD, obsessions in OCD, psychosis in schizophrenia, cognitive impairment in Alzheimer's disease, and migraine in migraineurs. The site of the anxiogenic action of mCPP is the hippocampus.[113] It also causes reduction in appetite which is not seen in CFS. I wonder whether the $5HT_{1c}$ receptor may be involved in the amelioration that immunosuppressive agents have on opioid withdrawal, perhaps mediated by a neuropeptide such as CRH. Could an action of the $5HT_{1c}$ receptor through the IL-1 receptor explain some effects of Ampligen not directly related to its effect on 2,5A synthetase/RNaseL?

Numerous peptides and proteins have serotonin binding sites which may modify their activity. These include GnRH, ACTH 4-10, and myelin basic protein. Muramyl dipeptide, important in slow-wave sleep induction, also binds to these sites, which are probably some, but not all, of the 5HT receptor subtypes. Glycopeptides such as muramyl dipeptide could have a neurotransmitter or hormonal function. The possibility exists that various peptides may mimic the function of 5-HT in normal physiology.[114] The implications of such a finding for PNI network theory have hardly been explored. The common report of CFS patients that they feel better (or worse) when taking antibiotics may relate to alteration of substances such as muramyl dipeptide produced by gut flora.

Treating the cognitive dysfunction of CFS is difficult. Although most patients have the usual encoding deficits of hippocampal dysfunction, some have more severe cognitive deficits to the degree that they could be diagnosed as having an amnestic disorder by DSM-III-R criteria. A perusal of the types of organic mental syndromes does not suggest any similar problem other than disorders which could impair the function of diencephalic and medial temporal structures. The cognitive dysfunction of CFS ("CFS dementia") may be treated by medication or by cognitive retraining.

CFS dementia is best treated by addressing the entire symptom complex. If a patient has a good response to treating fatigue and malaise, often the dementia will improve as well. Unfortunately, sometimes it will not. Next to fatigue, patients rate their CFS dementia as their worst symptom, since it so markedly impairs function. Little research has been done on cognitive enhancement in conditions other than Alzheimer dementia, but there is a priori reason to suspect that cognitive-enhancing agents, drugs that enhance cerebral metabolism ("nootropics"), might work better in CFS dementia, since there is probably little structural damage.[115] I have employed several strategies, but none has been very successful.

Augmenting cholinergic function with available agents has been somewhat effective, occasionally dramatically so. I use low doses of pyridostigmine (Mestinon) and/or transdermal nicotine patches. Patients may have increased mental clarity, more energy, anxiolysis, increased strength, cognitive enhancement, and even analgesia. Precursor loading with lecithin or choline has been ineffective, except to treat fasciculations. Selegiline HCl (Eldepryl), a MAOI with some cholinergic activity, has not been helpful, although it would be interesting to also give physostigmine or pilocarpine to stimulate post-synaptic cholinergic receptors. Synapton, a sustained release physostigmine, is in phase III trials. Tacrine HCl (Cognex), a cholinesterase inhibitor, is available for use under an investigational new drug application (IND) and would be interesting to try. It may be appropriate to test cholinergic function first, by means of a scopolamine challenge test. Linopirine, an agent that stimulates the release of acetylcholine, dopamine, and serotonin, is currently in phase III trials for SDAT and would also be an interesting drug to try. Acetyl-2-carnitine, a neuroprotective agent, is also in phase III trials. Its mechanism of action is unknown, but it may be an acetyl donor. Many of these drugs, and those to be mentioned subsequently, are currently being marketed in countries outside the United States.

Nerve growth factor (NGF) is a neurotrophic agent being investigated for senile dementia Alzheimer's type (SDAT) and Parkinson's disease. It may retard neuronal degeneration. NGF should be investigated further for safety before I would suggest trials in CFS dementia. NGF synthesis is stimulated by IL-1 beta and therefore levels of NGF might be reduced in CFS. NGF increases the density of dendritic spines.

My efforts to alter neurotransmitter levels have not been very

successful. My strategies to increase (or decrease) serotonin, glutamate, aspartate, somatostatin, CRH, substance P, opioids, norepinephrine, dopamine, and vasopressin have not worked. Various
agents to increase neuronal membrane fluidity have not helped,
either. Insulin-like growth factor 1 (IGF-1), another name for Somatomedin-C, is low in FM, and is being used in clinical trials. It
may be helpful in CFS/FM treatment.

Nootropic agents, as mentioned previously, may have helped
some patients. Piracetam, beneficial in dyslexia, may be of value, but
oxiracetam (Neuromet), available in Italy, may work better. Ergoloid
mesylates (Hydergine), even in high doses, have been disappointing
in CFS dementia. Vinpocetine (Ceractin) has been used in multi-infarct dementia. My two patients who have tried it reported no improvement in cognition. No one has tried gangliosides.

I am not aware of any research to suggest increased production of
beta-amyloid in CFS dementia, and would not advocate strategies
to block the production of amyloid precursor protein. Although
excitotoxins may play a role in CFS dementia, my attempts to
modulate them have not resulted in clinical improvement.

The most dramatic results in CFS dementia that I have seen have
been with IVIG, which often produces immediate results, but usually in the context of general symptomatic improvement. In CFS
patients with viral encephalopathy, killing the virus or blocking a
cytokine or a neurotoxic gene product would be the ideal treatments. The dementia is usually worse early in the illness, but a few
patients gradually deteriorate neurocognitively, even if other symptoms remain about the same, or even improve. CFS dementia, like
CFS itself, is not a unitary process. In the Ampligen experiment,
improvement in dementia was positively correlated with a decrease
in elevated levels of 2,5A synthetase/RNase L.[116] This result suggests either that immunotransmitters are etiologic, or that the antiviral activity of Ampligen could have reduced expression of gene
products. A major, if not the major, improvement in the Ampligen
study was in cognitive function.

There is almost nothing in the peer reviewed scientific literature
about the nature of cognitive dysfunction in CFS, and literally nothing about how to manage it. An issue of the *CFIDS Chronicle* (Physician's Forum, Volume I, Number 2, Fall 1991) was devoted to this

topic. Tarras Onischenko, PhD, discussed CFS dementia in the context of "diaschisis theory, the theoretical assumption that a temporary dysfunction due to a 'neuronal shock' in which edema, metabolic disturbance, and decreased blood perfusion all interfere with the nervous system and disrupt function until the CNS returns to more normal levels." This view, not unlike what I have described in this book, would account for the waxing and waning of CFS symptoms. Onischenko, as well as Curt Sandman, PhD, and Linda Miller Iger, PhD, describe mnemonic devices and strategies to improve cognition. Onischenko emphasizes that cognitive functioning is interrelated with emotional functioning, family-environmental demands, and social-behavioral functioning, and that all of these aspects should be addressed to produce the best outcome. Readers are referred to this journal for specific suggestions. My patients find cognitive rehabilitation to be very helpful, but it must be tailored to the individual. Some of them have been to hospital units which specialize in head trauma rehabilitation and have not been particularly improved.

CFS DEMENTIA TREATMENT

How, then, to understand and treat CFS dementia? If CFS is a multi-causal process, then the best therapy would involve the identification of the etiologic factors involved. A neurotoxic process is attractive, with perhaps an autoimmune organic mental syndrome in those whose self-antigens cross-react with viral antigens, or when superantigens are involved. The latter patients would have more severe dementia, and perhaps evidence of autoimmune processes elsewhere in the body. Neurotoxins, serotonin, and one or more hypothalamic peptides and their higher regulatory transmitters could be modulated. One would expect those with the most severe dementia to have the most UBOs on MRI and for these to be small areas of gliosis. Certain patients could have a very mild vasculitis, and a few could have demyelination. MRI scans show multiple punctate foci in the upper centrum ovale in midsaggital sections and in the high parasagittal white matter tracts. Bilateral focal areas of increased signal intensity are also seen in white matter tracts.[117] These findings differ from MRI reports of patients with severe depression.[118]

General treatment approaches would also reflect ideas regarding the limbic system developed in this book. Heteromodal inputs to limbic areas could be modified by cognitive-behavioral therapy and other techniques to modify behavioral state. It is well established that transmission to and from the limbic system is dependent on behavioral state,[119] and that short-term facilitation or inhibition of neuronal impulses can differ markedly with this variable. Behavioral state modulation of limbic neuronal transmission occurs very rapidly, and is best understood in electrophysiologic terms.[120] The neurochemistry of very rapid state changes is still rather obscure, but transmitters are known to change rapidly as states change, a phenomenon perhaps best studied in freely moving animals with implanted electrodes and cannulas. Thus the boundary between psychologic and organic etiology is more a matter of perspective, since every behavior must ultimately have an organic basis, unless the concept of a soul is invoked, as it was by Descartes to resolve his duality.

Antidepressants do not work only by altering levels of neurotransmitters, but also by changing arborization of dendrites.[121] Decreased dendritic arborization has been noted in a neonatal rat stress model of somatosensory amplification. Synapses in neuronal cultures exposed to tricyclics displayed increased numbers of synaptic vesicles and more extensive membrane specializations than in control cultures, and increased numbers of coated vesicles both pre- and post-synaptically. The density of apical dendritic spines on CA1 hippocampal neurons is directly related to estrogen concentrations in the normal estrus cycle of the adult female rat.[122] Thus synapse density can actually fluctuate in the normal adult mammalian brain. Lower density of dendritic spines could also be related to decreased levels of nerve growth factor and could represent a neuroanatomic cause for somatosensory amplification, if less dendritic arborization is correlated to imprecise modulation of sensory input. Such findings could also relate to late luteal phase dysphoria (LLPD), perhaps an example of somatosensory amplification. Patients with LLPD also develop panic attacks when challenged with lactate.[123] Most behavioral changes are mediated by synaptic plasticity and structural change, a process well demonstrated in learning.[124] Numerous neuronal and glial factors participate, and neuropharmacologic agents must alter levels of these substances as part of their mode of action. Sleep deprivation can be immunosuppressive. If one supposes that the alpha-EEG non-REM sleep abnormality is a form of sleep deprivation, it is possible, as is being currently investigated by Moldofsky, that IL-1, involved in sleep induction, may not have a proper central effect in CFS, or may not be secreted appropriately. An injection of IL-1 at the outset of sleep deprivation in rats prevented immunosuppression, but was immunosuppressive if given to sleeping rats. It would be interesting to test whether a rapid state change such as hypnosis could affect performance on cognitive testing in CFS. Although I see little evidence that implicates the pineal gland and melatonin secretion in CFS pathophysiology, the frequency of disturbances of biologic rhythm suggests a dysfunction. The alpha-EEG non-REM sleep abnormality may be a result of abnormal pineal function.[125] CFS patients may be more prone to seasonal affective disorder and sleep phase disorders, either phase advance (waking up earlier) or phase delay. Both types of problems may be treated with bright light therapy[126] which terminates melatonin secretion, thought to be inappropriate in many circadian disorders. Bright light therapy probably should be used more often in CFS. Cranial electrostimulation could also be of value, if done in an appropriate manner. The effect of magnetic fields on the brain should be considered if this form of therapy is to have maximum efficacy.[127]

Of the techniques to alter CNS neurotransmission by physical methods, acupuncture is probably the most widely used. This treatment is often fairly effective. Another strategy, not at all well known, is modulating trigeminal nerve activity.

TRIGEMINAL NERVE FUNCTION AND TREATMENT

The tryptamine derivative sumatriptan is an agonist at the $5HT_{1D}$ binding site. It contracts cerebral arteries and closes cerebral arteriovenous shunts. It has been thought that the mechanism of action was evidence for the "vasculogenic" theory of migraine. Recent research, however, does not support this hypothesis, particularly in the case of common migraine, and trigeminal nerve afferents producing a "sterile inflammation" around pial vessels as a means of pain production has gained more credibility. This response is suppressed by sumatriptan and other antimigraine drugs such as ergotamine.[128] It has been reported that most of the substance P surrounding pial blood vessels resides within afferent nerve fibers from trigeminal ganglion cells.[129] CGRP may be co-localized with the substance P.[130]

It may be that the cranial nerves, particularly the trigeminal, are involved in other disorders besides migraine headache, a condition which is common among CFS patients. Substance P-containing trigeminal sensory neurons project to the nucleus of the solitary tract and may alter vagal or glossopharyngeal sensory information.[131] IL-1 can induce substance P secretion. Acupuncture points of the head are most often used in CFS because the trigeminal nerve has extensive connections with the VII, VIII, IX, and X cranial nerves, C-2, and the autonomic nervous system, perhaps mediated in part by endogenous opioids and other neuropeptides found in the substantia gelatinosa.[132]

Numerous nerve branches in the vicinity of the temporomandibular joint distributed to the ear, temple, cheek, tongue, and teeth may be compressed in some patients with TMPDS and can simulate trigeminal neuralgia.[133] Trigeminal nerve afferents project to the reticular formation and thalamus and thus may have widespread effects. Proparacaine 0.5% ophthalmic solution in the ipsilateral eye can produce rapid and long-lasting treatment of trigeminal neuralgia[134] and atypical facial pain. Proparacaine is of value in cluster and hemicranial migraine headache and sometimes fibromyalgia. Other ophthalmic agents may also ameliorate CFS by modulating trigeminal input to limbic structures. I am currently investigating ocular adrenergic and muscarinic agonists and antagonists, as well as prostaglandin synthesis inhibitors to treat CFS. (See Appendix.)

Trigeminal nerve afferents also supply the tentorial nerves to the dura mater around the medial temporal lobes and the orbitofrontal cortex. This anatomical projection was used to explain why HSV-1, which is latent in the trigeminal ganglion, may infect limbic structures. More recently, of course, distinctive limbic receptors have been identified and are thought to explain the phenomenon more readily. Transneuronal spread from trigeminal nuclei to limbic-related nuclei such as the locus ceruleus and raphe has been postulated.

Trigeminal stimulation has produced excitability of vagus nuclear neurons in cats and can produce alterations in the transmission to the thoracic and abdominal viscera. There are also inputs from trigeminal cutaneous receptors to vagal nuclei in human volunteers which increase vagal cardiac outflow.

Parasympathetic fibers from the otic ganglion travel in the mandibular branch of the trigeminal nerve, and compression of these fibers could cause abnormalities of salivary gland secretion.

Horseradish peroxidase tracing of trigeminal nerve projections in monkeys shows a large projection to the ipsilateral ventral posteromedial nucleus of the thalamus (VPM), but also to the intralaminar nuclei in squirrel monkeys, a potential area for limbic innervation.

I have devoted this amount of space to the sensory trigeminal nerve in order to illustrate that there may be alternative measures such as a simple maxillary splint which might treat the symptoms of CFS in a non-invasive way not involving administration of drugs. We are investigating such a device. A nasal dilator has been reported to relieve chronic fatigue.[135]

Consideration of the regulation of the motor function of the trigeminal nerve, which innervates the muscles of mastication, yields insights into the possible pathophysiology of bruxism and TMPDS. Several papers over the last decade from the laboratory of M. Ohta in Kyushu, Japan,[136] and Gary Bobo[137] in Paris implicate the central amygdaloid nucleus in control of masseteric and myohyoid digastric function. The amygdaloid complex projects fibers to the brain stem, around the trigeminal motor nucleus, primarily on the ipsilateral side. It appears from Ohta's work that amygdaloid stimulation can excite neurons in the supratrigeminal area (STA) which projects to the contralateral trigeminal motor nucleus. Ohta concludes that "the shortest crossing amygdala-motoneuronal pathway is probably disynaptic and mediated by commisural STA neurons."

The possible role of the amygdala in the pathogenesis of TMPDS is compatible with the limbic hypothesis of CFS. TMPDS is very common in the general population, and even more common in the CFS population, in whom it is often a premorbid disorder. Although

I have often found it to be associated with mood disorders, many patients have severe bruxism with no past or family history of mood disorders. This may be a variant in limbic function, perhaps akin to panic disorder without panic.

PAIN MECHANISMS AND TREATMENT

Much of the research in pain mechanisms and treatment can be applied to CFS, since, like pain, "exhaustion," as discussed by Karpati,[138] is probably mediated by a CNS neural network with no single location. The neurobiology of pain is complex and poorly understood. A simplified model has been provided by Howard Fields, who divides pain into a sensory, an affective, and an evaluative component.[139] The sensory component results from activation of peripheral nociceptors and transmission through pain pathways to the ventrobasal thalamus, and then to the somatosensory cortex.

The affective component is activated by the same nociceptors but involves anatomical projections to the hypothalamus, limbic thalamus, frontal cortex, and classic limbic system.

The evaluative component is determined by the cognitive strategy of the individual patient. An example cited by Fields is whether a headache might be a sign of a brain tumor to someone. Thus somatizers would have altered cognitive strategies which would affect the evaluative process. Mood disorders would influence pain through the affective process.

A simplified pain circuit involves stimulation of a peripheral nociceptor, transmission through the spinothalamic and spinal reticulothalamic pathways, relayed from the thalamus to the frontal and somatosensory cortices. Pathways from the frontal cortex and hypothalamus activate cells in the midbrain, which control spinal pain transmission via cells in the pons and medulla.

As previously discussed, the periaqueductal gray region is a major outflow target of the limbic system, including the orbitofrontal cortex. Its main output is opioidergic, and it is a primary target for analgesia by brain stimulation.

For several years, Fields has been studying cells in the medulla called "on" cells and "off" cells.[140] When the off-cell fires, pain is inhibited, probably by an opioidergic mechanism. It is difficult for pain to be transmitted while the off-cell is firing. A pause in the off-cell permits pain to be transmitted. The on-cell has a facilitating effect on pain transmission. It becomes silent after morphine administration and fires at an even higher rate than baseline when morphine analgesia is reversed by naloxone. Narcotic withdrawal pain may be mediated by rebound facilitation of pain via increased firing of the on-cell. Fields concludes that there are facilitory as well as inhibitory components to pain modulation, and that pain can exist without peripheral noxious stimulation. Fields also indicates that pain transmission cells can fire without activation of nociceptors, a mechanism of "psychogenic pain." He wonders whether those persons prone to somatosensory amplification might inhibit the off-cells and activate the on-cells. I wonder whether chronic pain syndromes may be characterized by a deficiency of CRH or IL-1, which increases nociceptive thresholds.

Much of our understanding of the role of the limbic system in pain derives from the use of limbic surgery in the treatment of intractable pain. To summarize the results of the last 50 years: the best results have been obtained with bilateral anterior cingulotomy in a patient who is anxious and/or depressed and in whom antidepressant and/or anticonvulsant medication is maintained. Cingulotomy may help patients when deep brain stimulation does not. Somatoform disorders, personality disorders, and primary substance abuse were among the exclusionary criteria for such surgery at Massachusetts General Hospital in 1987.[141]

The cingulate gyrus, as one of the paralimbic structures, connects with all other areas of the expanded definition of the limbic system, as well as the heteromodal association areas, which are primarily in the frontal lobes. Cingulotomy severs connections between these various structures to a significant extent. This surgery is also used to relieve intractable anxiety and depression, but post-operative personality change does not correlate with pain relief.

Neurochemical changes subsequent to cingulotomy are still poorly understood, but an opioidergic mechanism must be involved. Patients addicted to narcotics do not have withdrawal symptoms after cingulotomy for intractable pain. It is tempting to speculate that there is a direct connection between the anterior cingulate (or related structures) and the off-cells of Fields. Bilateral injections of morphine into the corticomedial amygdala produce analgesic effects in certain experimental paradigms. Serotoninergic fibers are implicated in pain modulatory circuits involving the amygdala, nucleus accumbens, and the habenula. I wonder whether such fibers are affected by ritanserin, the $5HT_2/5HT_{1c}$ antagonist which ameliorates FM and also blocks opioid withdrawal.

Endogenous pain control substances include the opioids: endorphins, enkephalins, and dynorphins; biogenic amines: serotonin, dopamine, and norepinephrine; neuropeptides: substance P and other tachykinins, somatostatin, bombesin, and possibly CGRP, TRH, and ACTH; acetylcholine; adenosine; GABA; calcitonin, neurotensin, eicosanoids, and histamine.[142] Most of these agents have been studied in the brain stem and spinal cord, but few in the limbic system.

I have tried to pharmacologically alter the regulation of the above substances in every way I know in the treatment of FM, and there is no one effective treatment for patients. Some of them work through opioidergic mechanisms, while others do not. Some enhance pain, others inhibit it. Either the neural network regulation of FM pain is too heterogeneous between patients (many of whom have also had cognitive behavioral therapy), or there is a unifying neurochemical derangement which has not been detected or addressed (perhaps involving IL-1). It may be worthwhile to use agonists and antagonists for the above substances as pharmacologic probes in the treatment of the patient with severe FM who has not responded to the usual treatment trials: heterocyclic antidepressants, fluoxetine, cyclobenzaprine, H-2 blockers, NSAIDs, and alprazolam. Some of my patients, especially those with severe headaches, respond exceptionally well to somatostatin octreotide (Sandostatin) in a dose of 0.05 mg SQ once or twice a day. Often only headache is relieved, but sometimes all symptoms are. I am investigating how these patients may differ from Sandostatin non-responders. These may be patients with decreased, rather than increased, activity of IL-beta antagonists, since somatostatin is a substance P antagonist, and substance P increases concentration of IL-1 beta.[143] Multidisciplinary treatment, including psychotherapy, stress reduction, exercise modification, and trigger-point therapy, when added to drugs works considerably better than drugs used alone. If Ampligen indeed proves to be a "magic bullet" for many patients, this outcome could be altered. My preliminary observations suggest that most patients with FM respond well to low dose nitroglycerin and/or transdermal nicotine patches. A controlled experiment with Ismael Mena, MD, is pending (see Conclusion).

ALTERNATIVE CFS TREATMENTS

There are a large number of nutritional, or "alternative" (holistic) treatments for CFS. I have not found most of them to be very helpful. Among those that I have used with some success is intravenous vitamin C (sodium ascorbate), in doses of 25-50 grams, diluted in normal saline, with calcium gluconate added (because ascorbate in high doses is a calcium chelator) and magnesium sulfate to prevent magnesium shifts when calcium is added. I must admit that I thought IV ascorbate was quackery when I first heard about it. After numerous patients had extolled its virtues, however, I decided to try it. The treatment seemed safe, and CFS, if it was a disorder of immune activation, could generate destructive free radicals which could cause tissue damage. After we began to do brain SPECT scans and saw patients with degrees of hypoperfusion that were in the ischemic range, it also became possible that free radicals could be generated as a result of lipid peroxidation and other mechanisms previously discussed. Furthermore, when a CFS-associated viral agent was found to possibly be a retrovirus, credence was lent to the use of IV ascorbate because vitamin C inhibited HIV infection of cultured cells, although HIV transcription was not blocked.[144] The mechanism was unknown, although it was said that supra-physiologic levels of ascorbate would be needed to have this effect, levels which could only be achieved by the intravenous route.

Patients with HIV have glutathione deficiencies, and the drug N-acetyl-cysteine, which replenishes glutathione, has been used in AIDS (and CFS). Its effect in AIDS is to slow HIV production by inhibiting viral transcription. N-acetyl-cysteine has been tried sporadically in CFS, but the results have not been remarkable. Newborn rats with drug-induced glutathione deficiency developed multiple organ failure unless treated with very high levels of ascorbate. Massive doses of ascorbate may actually be the source of high energy electrons used in the process of free radical scavenging and may achieve this process independently of the electron transport chain consisting of NADH or NADPH$\rightarrow$FADH$_2\rightarrow$ GSH. Since the human body cannot synthesize vitamin C, as many animals do, it is dependent on the re-reduction of free radical scavengers such as ascorbate which donate their electrons, and there is a limit to this system. I have used other free radical scavengers in CFS, such as vitamin E, selenium, beta-carotene, etc., but I never saw any effect. I was surprised when I first gave IV ascorbate and saw patients improve, since I had previously thought it was a difficult and expensive way to give a placebo. I usually tried it on patients who failed to respond to other treatments, especially ranitidine, doxepin, and fluoxetine, but many patients had seen over ten physicians prior to seeing me and had tried numerous other therapies without relief. Those who responded to IV ascorbate (oral ascorbate, even to "bowel tolerance," did not help much), felt generally improved for several days to several weeks. Approximately 50% of my patients were improved with IV ascorbate, half of these markedly. High dose oral vitamin C, 60 mg/kg, has been reported to enhance NK function in normal subjects,[145] and also does so in CFS patients.[146] There is no significant symptomatic improvement accompanying the increase in NK function, which suggests that the NK functional deficit is an epiphenomenon.

The list of treatments my patients have tried with the cooperation of the AIDS underground is long. It includes a mistletoe extract called Iscador; a milk thistle extract, silymarin; Artemesia annua; glycyrrhizin; and coenzyme Q-10, a necessary co-factor in mitochondrial oxidative phosphorylation. Coenzyme Q-10 is readily available in health food stores and has some appeal since Behan has suggested for several years that there are mitochondrial abnormalities in CFS. He has recently published biopsy results to demonstrate this finding.[147] Coenzyme Q-10 has been reported to prevent the progression of dementia in two patients with Alzheimer's disease.[148] A mitochondrial process is attractive in CFS pathophysiology and would synergize in the purported reduction of ATP caused by increased 2,5A/RNase L activity. Muscle biopsies in my patients have not revealed mitochondrial abnormalities. Mitochondrial mRNA has not been tested, but it is possible that a CNS mitochondrial deficit is present in CFS patients. L-carnitine, another substance involved in mitochondrial function, may have helped some of my patients.

Some patients respond well to homeopathic remedies. This form of treatment prescribes extremely small quantities of substances to which a patient is thought to be reactive. It is possible that the technique alters the sensitivity of dysregulated limbic receptors.

Other treatments to be considered are removal of mercury amalgams from teeth or of silicone implants. There are no diagnostic tests to see whether these substances are causing an immune derangement, and it is possible that those patients who have adverse reactions may have a limbic vulnerability to do so. If there is is an abnormality in peripheral immunotransmitters, it has not yet been detected. I have seen dramatic improvement in two patients who elected silicone explantation. A double-blind procedure, or sham operation, would be ethically difficult to do in such patients in order to minimize the placebo effect.

REFERENCES

1. Lloyd AR, Hickie I, Wakefield D, Boughton C, Dwyer AM. A double-blind, placebo-controlled trial of intravenous immunoglobulin therapy in patients with chronic fatigue syndrome: a double-blind placebo-controlled trial. *Am J Med* 89: 561-568, 1990.

2. Peterson P, Shepard J, Macres M, et al. Controlled trial of intravenous immunoglobulin in chronic fatigue syndrome. *Am J Med* 89: 554-560, 1990.

3. Jessop C. Presented at CFIDS: Unraveling the mystery, Charlotte NC, November 18, 1990.

4. Galland L. The effect of systemic microbes on systemic immunity. In: Jenkins R and Mowbray JF (eds.). *Postviral Fatigue Syndrome,* Chichester, John Wiley, 1991.

5. Levitt P. A monoclonal antibody to limbic system neurons. *Science* 223:229-231,1984.

6. Newman NJ, Bell IR, McHee AC. Paraneoplastic limbic encephalitis. *Biol Psychiatry* 27:529-542,1990.

7. Damasio AR, van Hoesen GW. The limbic system and the localization of herpes simplex encephalitis. *J Neurol Neurosurg Psychiatry* 48:297-301, 1985.

8. Ludwig H, Bode L, Gosztony, G. Borna disease: a persistent virus infection of the central nervous system. *Prog Med Virol* 35:107-151, 1988.

9. Amsterdam JD, Winokur A, Dyson W. Borna disease virus: a possible etiologic factor in human affective disorders? *Arch Gen Psychiatry* 42: 1093-1096, 1985.

10. Lavi E, Fisman PS, Highkin MH. Limbic encephalitis after inhalation of a murine coronavirus. *Lab Invest* 58(1): 31-36, 1988.

11. Oldstone MBA. Viral alteration of cell function. *Sci Am* 261(2): 42-49, 1989.

12. McVaugh W, Lawrence B, Kulkarni A, Pizzini R, Van Buren C, Rudolph F, Wolinsky I, DaFay N. Suppression of opiate withdrawal by cyclosporin A and dietary modification. *Life Sci* 44: 977-983, 1989.

13. Berthold H, Borel JF, Fluckigor E. Enigmatic action of ciclosporine A on the naloxone-precipitated morphine withdrawal syndrome in mice. *Neuroscience* 31(1): 97-103, 1989.

14. Bouckoms AJ. Psychosurgery for pain. In: Wall PD and Melzack R. (eds). *Textbook of Pain*. Edinburgh, Churchill Livingstone, 1989.

15. Webster EC, Tracey DE, DeSouza EB. Upregulation of interleukin-1 receptors in mouse AtT-20 pituitary tumor cells following treatment with corticotropin-releasing factor. *Endocrinology* 129(5): 2796-2798, 1991.

16. Muller H, Hammer E, Heim KE, Hess G. Interferon-alpha-2-induced stimulation of ACTH and cortisol secretion in man. *Neuroendocrinology* 54: 499-503, 1991.

17. Baron S, Tyring SK, Fleischmann WR, Coppenhaver DH, Niegel DW, Kimpel GR, Stanton GJ, Hughes TK. The interferons: mechanisms of action and clinical applications. *JAMA* 266(10): 1375-1383, 1991.

18. Mezey E, Palkovits M. Localization of targets for anti-ulcer drugs in cells of the immune system. *Science* 258:1662-1665, 1992.

19. Falus A, Meretey K. Histamine: an early messenger in inflammatory and immune reactions. *Immunol Today* 13(5): 154-156, 1992.

20. Linde A, Andersson B, Svenson SB, Ahrne H, Carlsson M, Forsberg P, Hugo H, Korstorp A, Lenkel R, Lindwall A, Luflenius A, Sall C, Anderson J. Serum levels of lymphokines and soluble cellular receptors in primary Epstein-Barr virus infection and in patients with chronic fatigue syndrome. *J Infect Dis* 165: 994-1000, 1992.

21. Lloyd AR, Hickie I, Wakefield D, Boughton C, Dwyer AM. A double-blind, placebo-controlled trial of intravenous immunoglobulin therapy in patients with chronic fatigue syndrome: a double-blind placebo-controlled trial. *Am J Med* 89: 561-568, 1990.

22. Kalkman HO, Fozard JR. 5HT receptor subtypes and their role in disease. *Curr Opinion Neurol Neurosurg* 4: 560-565, 1991.

23. Imbach P (ed.). *Immunotherapy with Intravenous Immunoglobulins*. London, Academic Press, 1991.

24. Pouplard AGF, Bottazo D, Doniach D, Roitt IV. Binding of human immunoglobulins to pituitary ACTH cells. *Nature* 261: 142-144, 1976.

25. Steinbach TL, Hermann WJ. The treatment of CFIDS with Kutapressin. *CFIDS Chronicle*, pp 25-30, Spring/Summer 1990.

26. Suzuki M, Higuchi S, Tako Y, Taki S, Miwa K, Hamuro J. Induction of endogenous lymphokine-activated killer activity by combined administration of lentinan and interleukin 2. *Int J Immunopharmacol* 12(6): 613-623, 1990.

27. Spinedi E, Hadid R, Daneva T, Gaillard R. Cytokines stimulate the CRH but not the vasopressin neuronal system: evidence for a median eminence site of interleukin-6 action. *Neuroendocrinology* 56: 46-53, 1992.

28. Lloyd A, Hickie I, Brockman A, Hickie C, Wilson A, Dwyer J, Wakefield D. A controlled trial of immunological and congnitive-behavioral therapy for patients with chronic fatigue syndrome. *Am J Med* 1992 (in press).

29. Solomon G. Personal communication, 1992.

30. Renoux G, Renoux M. Imuthiol, a specific immunopotentiator. *Int J Immunotherapy* VI (1): 25-35, 1990.

31. Flechas J. Personal communication, 1992.

32. Parker LN. *Adrenal Androgens in Clinical Medicine.* Academic Press, San Diego, 1989.

33. Deutsch SI, Mastropaolo J, Hitri A. GABA-active steroids: endogenous modulators of GABA-gated chloride ion conductance. *Clin Neuropharmacol* 15(5): 352-364, 1992.

34. Paul SM, Purdy RH. Neuroactive steroids. FASEB J 3: 647-654, 1992.

35. Hu ZY, Borreau E, Jung-Testas I, Robel P, Baulieu E-E. Neurosteroids: oligodendrocyte mitochondria convert cholesterol to prognenolene. *Proc Natl Acad Sci USA* 88: 4553-4557, 1987.

36. Corpechot C, Robel P, Axelson M, Sjovall J, Baulieu E-E. Characterization and measurement of dehydroepiandrosterone sulfate in rat brain. *Proc Natl Acad Sci* USA 78: 4704-4707, 1981.

37. Crowley JN, Glowa JR, Majowska MD, Paul SM. Anxiolytic activity of an endogenous adrenal steroid. *Brain Res* 398: 382-385, 1986.

38. Kare M. Direct pathways to the brain. *Science* 163: 952-953, 1968.

39. Behan PO, Behan WMW, Horrobin DF. A placebo-controlled trial of n-3 and n-6 essential fatty acids in the treatment of post-viral fatigue syndrome. *Acta Neurol Scand* 82: 209-216, 1990.

40. Good RA, Lorenz E. Nutrition and cellular immunity. *Int J Immunopharmacol* 14(3): 361-366, 1992.

41. Simon HB. Exercise and human immune function. In: Ader R, Felten DF, and Cohen N. (eds.). *Psychoneuroimmunology,* second edition, San Diego, Academic Press, 1991.

42. Goldstein JA. Presented at: Chronic Fatigue Syndrome and the Brain, Bel Air, CA, April 24-26, 1992.

43. Mathias JR, Ferguson KL, Clench MH. Debilitating "functional" bowel disease controlled by leuprolide acetate, gonadotropin-releasing hormone (GnRH) analog. *Dig Dis Sci* 34(5): 761-766, 1989.

44. McGrail M, et al. Peptide T studies: Neurophysiologic results. VII Intl Conf AIDS, Florence. Vol 1:194 (M.B. 2049), 1991.

45. Buzy J, Brenneman DE, Pert CB, Martin A, Salazar A, Ruff MR. Potent gp-120-like neurotoxic activity in the cerebrospinal fluid is blocked by peptide T. *Brain Res* 598:10-18, 1992.

46. Brenneman D. Neuroimmune interactions: implications for neuro-AIDS and neurodevelopment. Presented at The Seminar in Behavioral Neuroimmunology, Los Angeles, UCLA School of Medicine, November 2, 1992.

47. Bredt DS, Snyder SH. Nitric oxide, a novel neuronal messenger. *Neuron* 8: 3-11, 1992.

48. Artzimovich N. Personal communication, 1992.

49. Demitrack MA, Greden JF. Chronic fatigue syndrome: The need for an integrative approach (editorial). *Biol Psychiatry* 30:747-752,1991.

50. Krishnan KRR, Doraiswamy PM, Venkataraman S, Reed DA, Richie JC. Current concepts in hypothalamo-pituitary-adrenal axis regulation. In: *Stress, Neuropeptides and Systemic Disease.* McCubbin JA, Kaufmann PG, Nemeroff CF (eds.). San Diego, Academic Press, 1991.

51. Borden N, Pepin M-C, Pfeiffer A. The mechanism of action of antidepressants on the hypothalamic-pituitary-adrenal axis may not be related to their effects on catecholamine uptake. *Neuroendocrinol Lett* 13(3): 208(abs), 1991.

52. Glowa JR, Bacher JD, Herkenham M, Gold PW. Selective anorexigenic effects of corticotropin releasing hormone in the rhesus monkey. *Prog Neuropsychopharmacol Biol Psychiatry* 15: 379-391, 1991.

53. Yehuda R, Giller EL, Southwick SM, Lowy MT, Mason JW. Hypothalamic-pituitary-adrenal dysfunction in post traumatic stress disorder. *Biol Psychiatry* 30: 1031-1048, 1991.

54. de Souza EB. CRH defects in Alzheimer's and other neurologic diseases. *Hosp Practice* 23(9): 59-76, 1988.

55. Geracioti TD, Orth DN, Ekhator NN, Blumenkopf B, Loosen PT. Serial cerebrospinal fluid corticotropin releasing hormone concentrations in healthy and depressed humans. *J Clin Endocrinol Metab* 74(6): 1325-1330, 1992.

56. Wessely S. Are there symptoms of low blood pressure? *Hosp Practice* 26(9A): 8-13, 1991.

57. Drummond PD. Disturbances in ocular sympathetic function and cerebral blood flow in unilateral migraine headache. *J Neurol Neurosurg Psychiatry* 53: 121-125, 1990.

58. Ewing DJ. Clinical aspects of primary and secondary autonomic failure. *Curr Opin Neurol Neurosurg* 4: 539-544, 1991.

59. Mathias JR. Personal communication, 1992.

60. Spyer KM. Physiology of the autonomic nervous system: CNS control of the cardiovascular system. *Curr Opin Neurol and Neurosurg* 4: 528-538, 1991.

61. Appenzeller O. *The Autonomic Nervous System: An Introduction to Basic and Clinical Concepts,* 4th Ed. New York: Elsevier, 1990.

62. Wessely S, Butler S, Chalder T, David A. The cognitive-behavioral management of the post-viral fatigue syndrome. In: *Post-viral Fatigue Syndrome,* Jenkins R and Mowbray JF (eds.). Chichester, Churchill Livingstone, 1991.

63. Lipowski ZJ. Somatization: the concept and its clinical application. *Am J Psychiatry* 145: 1358-1368, 1988.

64. Schacter S. Cognition and peripheralist-centralist controversies in motivation and emotion. In: Gazzaniga MS, Blakemore C (eds.): *Handbook of Psychobiology.* New York: Academic Press, 1975.

65. Simon GE, Von Korff M. Somatization and psychiatric disorder in the NIMH epidemiologic catchment area study. *Am J Psychiatry* 148(11): 1494-1500, 1991.

66. Abbey SE, Garfinkel PE. Neurasthenia and chronic fatigue syndrome: the role of culture in making a diagnosis. *Am J Psychiatry* 148(12): 1638-1646,1991.

67. Shorter E. *From Paralysis to Fatigue: A History of Psychosomatic Illness in the Modern Era.* New York, The Free Press, 1992.

68. Bass CM (ed.). *Somatization: Physical Symptoms and Psychological Illness.* Oxford, Blackwell Scientific Publications, 1990.

69. Bass CM, Gardner G. Hyperventilation syndrome. In Bass CM (ed.). *Somatization: Physical Symptoms and Psychological Illness.* Oxford, Blackwell Scientific Publications, 1990.

70. Lindsay S, Saqi S, Bass C. The test-retest reliability of the hyperventilation provocation test. *J Psychosomatic Res* 35(2/3): 155-162, 1991.

71. Harper RM. Neurophysiology of sleep. In: *Hypoxia, exercise and altitude: Proceedings of the Third Banff International Hypoxia Symposium.* New York, Alan R Liss, 65-73, 1991.

72. Baxter LR, Schwartz JM, Bergman KS, Szuba MP, Guze BH, Mazziotta, JC, Alazraki A, Selin CE, Ferng H-K, Munford P, Phelps ME. Caudate nucleus metabolic rate changes with both drug and behavior therapy for obsessive-compulsive disorder. *Arch Gen Psychiatry* 49: 681-689, 1992.

73. Reiman EM, Fosselman MJ, Fox PT, Raichle ME. Neuroanatomical correlates of anticipatory anxiety. *Science* 243: 1071-1073, 1989.

74. Drevets WC, Videem TO, MacLeod AH, Haller JW, Raichle ME. PET images of blood flow changes during anxiety: correction. *Science* 256: 1696, 1992.

75. Fesler FA. Valproate in combat-related posttraumatic stress disorder. *J Clin Psychiatry* 52: 361-364, 1991.

76. Brus I, and Wallack J. Phenelzine sulfate for chronic fatigue syndrome (abstr). *Gen Hosp Psych* 13(6): 366, 1991.

77. Bass CM (ed). *Somatization: Physical Symptoms and Psychological Illness.* Oxford, Blackwell Scientific Publications, 1990.

78. Wood PL, Rao TS. Morphine stimulation of mesolimbic and mesocortical but not nigrostriatal dopamine release in the rat as reflected by changes in 3-methosyltyramine levels. *Neuropharmacology* 30(4): 399-401, 1991.

79. Liebowitz MR, Quitkin FM, Stewart JW, McGrath PH, Harrison WM, Markowitz JS, Rabkin JG, Tricamo E, Goetz DM, Klein DF. Antidepressant specificity in atypical depression. *Arch Gen Psychiatry* 45: 129-138, 1988.

80. Mercier MA, Steward JW, Quitkin FM. A pilot sequential study of cognitive therapy and pharmacotherapy of atypical depression. *J Clin Psychiatry* 53: 166-170, 1992.

81. Post RM, Rubinow DR, Balenger JC. Conditioning, sensitization, and kindling: implications for the course of affective illness. In: *Neurobiology of Mood Disorders.* Post RM, Ballenger JC (eds.). Baltimore, Williams and Wilkins, 1984.

82. Post RM. Transduction of psychosocial stress into the neurobiology of recurrent affective disorder. *Am J Psychiatry* 149(8): 999-1010, 1992.

83. Brown MR. Neuropeptide-mediated regulation of the neuroendocrine and autonomic response to stress. In: *Stress, Neuropeptides, and Systemic Disease.* McCubbin JA, Haufmann PO, Nemeroff CB (eds). San Diego, Academic Press, 1991.

84. Martin JB, Reichlin S. *Clinical Neuroendocrinology*, edition 2. Philadelphia, FA Davis, 1987.

85. Russell IJ. Presented at: Chronic Fatigue Syndrome and the Brain, Bel Air, CA, April 24-26, 1992.

86. Demitrack MA, Gold PW, Dale JK, Krahn DD, Kling MA, Straus SE. Plasma and cerebrospinal monoamine metabolism in patients with chronic fatigue syndrome : preliminary findings. *Biol Psychiatry* 32 : 1065-1077, 1992.

87. Gorman JM, Liebowitz MR, Figer AJ, Stein J. A neuroanatomical basis for panic disorder. *Am J Psychiatry* 146(2): 148-161, 1989.

88. Caplan JD, Sharma T, Rosenblum LA, Friedman S, Bassoff TB, Barbour RL, Gorman JM. Effects of sodium lactate infusion on cisternal lactate and carbon dioxide levels in nonhuman primates. *Am J Psychiatry* 149(10): 1369-1373, 1992.

89. Mathew RJ, Wilson H. Anxiety and cerebral blood flow. *Am J Psychiatry* 147(7): 838-849, 1990.

90. Goldstein JA. Calcium channel blockers in the treatment of panic disorder. *J Clin Psychiatry* 46(12): 546, 1985.

91. Klein E, Uhde TW. Controlled study of verapamil for treatment of panic disorder. *Am J Psychiatry* 145: 431-434, 1988.

92. Gross PM, Zochodne DW, Wainman DS, Ho LT, Espinosa FJ, Weaver DF. Intraventricular endothelin-1 uncouples the blood flow: metabolism relationship in periventricular structures of the rat brain: involvement of L-type calcium channels. *Neuropeptides* 22: 155-165, 1992.

93. Gross PM, Wainman DS, Espinosa FJ, Mag S, Weaver DF. Cerebral hypermetabolism produced by intraventricular endothelin-1 in rats: inhibition by nimodipine. *Neuropeptides* 21: 211-223, 1992.

94. Gibbs DM. Hyperventilation-induced cerebral ischemia in panic disorder and the effect of nimodipine. *Am J Psychiatry* 149: 1589-1591, 1992.

95. Kolb H, Kolb-Bachofen V. Nitric oxide: a pathogenetic factor in autoimmunity. *Immunol Today* 32(5): 157-159, 1992.

96. Snyder SH, Bredt DS. Biological roles of nitric oxide. *Sci American:* 68-77, May 1992.

97. Meldrum B, Garthwaite J. EAA pharmacology: excitatory amino acid neurotoxicity and neurodegenerative disease. *Trends Pharmacol Sci* 11(9): 379-386, 1990.

98. Dawson TM, Bredt DS, Foktuhi M, Hwang PM, Snyder SH. Nitric oxide synthase and neuronal NADPH diaphorase are identical in brain and peripheral tissues. *Proc Natl Acad Sci USA,* 88: 7797-7801, 1991.

99. Faraci FM, Breese KR. Neuronally-derived nitric-oxide may mediate vasodilatation during increased neuronal activity in brain (meeting abstr). *Circulation* 86(4): 14, 1992.

100. Raszkiewicz JL, Linville DG, Kerwin JF, Wagenaar F, Arneric SP. Nitric oxide synthase is critical in mediating basal forebrain regulation of cortical cerebral circulation. *J Neurosci Res* 33: 129-135, 1992.

101. Nathan C. Nitric oxide as a secretory product of mammalian cells. *FASEB* 6: 3051-3064.

102. Lowenstein CJ, Snyder SH. Nitric oxide, a novel biological messenger. *Cell* 70: 705-707, 1992.

103. Girgis M. Biochemical patterns in limbic system circuitry: biochemical-electrophysiological interactions displayed by chemitrode techniques. In: *The Limbic System: Functional Organization and Clinical Disorders,* Raven Press, New York, pp. 55-56, 1986.

104. Rosenthal NE, Cameron CL. Exaggerated sensitivity to an organophosphate pesticide (letter). *Am J Psychiatry* 148(2): 270, 1991.

105. Schottfeld R. Workers with multiple chemical sensitivities: a psychiatric approach to diagnosis and treatment. In: Workers with multiple chemical sensitivities, Cullen MR (ed.), *Occup Med: State Art Rev* 2(4): 739-754, 1987.

106. Kandel ER, Hawkins RD. The biological basis of learning and individuality. *Sci American,* 267(3): 79-86, 1992.

107. Meldrum B, Garthwaite J. EAA pharmacology: excitatory amino acid neurotoxicity and neurodegenerative disease. *Trends Pharmacol Sci* 11(9): 379-386, 1990.

108. Tortella FC, Pellicano M, Bowery NG. Dextromethorphan and neuromodulation: old drug coughs up new activities. *Trends Pharmacol Sci* 10: 501-507, 1989.

109. Goldstein JA. Presented at: Chronic Fatigue Syndrome and Fibromyalgia: Pathophysiology and Treatment. Los Angeles, CA, 1990.

110. Kamoli P, Stansfield SC, Ashton CH, Hammond GL, Emanuel MB, Rawlins MD. Absence of withdrawal effects of ritanserin following chronic dosing in healthy volunteers. *Psychopharmacology* 108: 213-217, 1992.

111. Kapur S, Mann JJ. Role of the dopaminergic system in depression. *Biol Psychiatry* 32: 1-17, 1992.

112. Devaud LL, Hollingsworth EG, Cooper BR. Alterations in extracellular and tissue levels of biogenic amines in rat brain induced by the serotonin$_2$ receptor antagonist, ritanserin. *J Neurochem* 59(4): 1459-1466, 1992.

113. Kalkman HO, Fozard JR. 5HT receptor subtypes and their role in disease. *Curr Op Neurol Neurosurg* 4: 560-565, 1991.

114. Root-Bernstein RS, Westall FC. Serotonin binding sites. II. Muramyl dipeptide binds to serotonin binding sites on myelin basic protein, CHRH, and MSH-ACTH 4-10. *Brain Res Bull* 25: 827-841, 1990.

115. Sarter M. Taking stock of cognition enhancers. *Trends Pharmacol Sci* 12(12): 456-461, 1991.

116. Suhadolnik R. Personal communication, 1992.

117. Buchwald D, Cheney PR, Peterson DL, Henry B, Wormsley SB, Geiger A, Ablashi DR, Salhuddin Z, Saxinger C, Biddle R, Kikinis R, Jolesz FA, Folks T, Balachandran N, Peter JB, Gallo RC, Komaroff AL. A chronic illness characterized by fatigue, neurologic and immunologic disorders, and active human herpesvirus type 6 infection. *Ann Int Med* 116(2): 103-113, 1992.

118. Brown FW, Lewine RJ, Hudgins PA, Risch SC. White matter hyperintensity signals in psychiatric and non-psychiatric subjects. *Am J Psychiatry* 149(5): 620-625, 1992.

119. Austin KB, Bronzino JD, Morgane PJ. Paired-pulse facilitation and inhibition in the dentate gyrus is dependent on behavioral state. *Brain Res* 17(3): 594-604, 1989.

120. Tang C-M, Shi Q-Y, Katchman A, Lynch G. Modulation of the time course of fast EPSCSs and glutamate channel kinetics by aniracetam. *Science* 254: 288-290, 1991.

121. Azmitia EC, Whitaker-Azmitia PM, Awakening the sleeping giant: anatomy and plasticity of the brain serotoninergic system. *J Clin Psychiatry* 52(Suppl): 4-16, 1991.

122. Woolley CS, McEwen BS. Estradiol mediates fluctuation in hippocampal synapse density during the estrous cycle in the adult rat. *J Neurosci* 12(7): 2549-2554, 1992.

123. Facchinetti F, Romano G, Fava M, Genazzani AR. Lactate infusion induces panic attacks in patients with premenstrual syndrome. *Psychosom Med* 54: 288-296, 1992.

124. Massicote G, Baudry M. Triggers and substrates of hippocampal plasticity. *Neurosci Biobehav Rev* 15: 415-423, 1991.

125. Sandyk R. Alpha rhythm and the pineal gland. *Intern J Neuroscience* 63: 221-227, 1992.

126. Czeisler CA, Kronover RE, Allen JS, et al. Bright light induction of strong (type O) resetting of the human circadian pacemaker. *Science* 244: 1328-1333, 1989.

127. Sandyk R, Anninos PA, Tsagas N, Derpapas K. Magnetic fields in the treatment of Parkinson's disease. *Intern J Neuroscience* 63: 141-150, 1992.

128. Humphrey PPA, Feniuk W. Mode of action of the anti-migraine drug sumatriptan. *Trends Pharmacol Sci* 12: 444-445, 1991.

129. Liu-Chen L-Y, Han DH, Moskowitz MA. Pia arachnoid contains substance P originating from trigeminal neurons. *Neuroscience* 9(4): 803-808, 1983.

130. Uddman R, Edvinsson L, Ekman R, Kingman T, McCulloch J. Innervation of the feline cerebral vasculature by nerve fibers containing calcitonin gene-re-

lated peptide: trigeminal origin and co-existence with substance P. *Neurosci Letters* 62: 131-136, 1988.

131. South EH, Ritter RC. Substance P-containing trigeminal sensory neurons project to the nucleus of the solitary tract. *Brain Res* 372: 283-289, 1986.

132. Shokljev A, Koruga E. The role of the trigeminal nerve in acupuncture. *Acupuncture Electro-therapeutics Res Int* J 13: 67-78, 1988.

133. Zavonik MK, Fichte CM. Trigeminal neuralgia relieved by ophthalmic anesthetic. *JAMA* 265:2807, 1991.

134. Ohta M. Amygdaloid and cortical facilitation or inhibition of trigeminal motoneurons in the rat. *Brain Res* 291: 39-48, 1984.

135. Chester AC. Chronic fatigue relieved by a nasal dilator. *Am J Otolaryngol* 14(1)71, 1993.

136. Ohta M, Moriyama Y. Supratrigeminal neurons mediate the shortest disynaptic pathway from the central amygdaloid nucleus to the contralateral trigeminal motoneurone in the rat. *Science* 253: 555-557, 1991.

137. Bobo EG, Bonvallet M. Amygdala and masseteric reflex: I. Facilitation, inhibition, and diphasic modifications of the reflex, induced by localized amygdaloid stimulation. *Electroenceph Clin Neurophysiol* 39: 329-339, 1975.

138. Karpati G. Presented at: Workshop on research directions for myalgic encephalomyelitis/chronic fatigue syndrome, Vancouver, Canada, May 11, 1991.

139. Fields H. Depression and pain: a neurobiological model. *Neuropsychiat, Neuropsychol, Behav Neurol* 4(1): 83-92, 1991.

140. Fields HL, Morgan MM. Activity of nociceptive modulatory neurons in the rostral ventromedial medulla associated with volume expansion-induced antinociception. *Pain* 52(1):1-10, 1993.

141. Bouckoms AJ. Psychosurgery for pain. In: Wall PD and Melzack R (eds.). *Textbook of Pain*. Edinburgh, Churchill Livingstone, 1989.

142. Yaksh TL, Almone LD. The central pharmacology of pain treatment. In: Wall PD, Merck R (eds.). *Textbook of Pain*, Edinburgh, Churchill Livingstone, 1989.

143. Martin FC, Charles AC, Sanderson MJ, Merrill JE. Substance P stimulates IL-1 production by astrocytes via intracellular calcium. *Brain Res* 599:13-18, 1992.

144. Cathcart RF. A unique function for ascorbate. *Med Hypothes* 35: 32-37, 1991.

145. Vojdani A. Submitted for publication, 1992.

146. Vojdani A. Personal communication, 1992.

147. Behan WMH, More IAR, Behan PO. Mitochondrial abnormalities in the postviral fatigue syndrome. *Acta Neuropath* 83: 61-65, 1991.

148. Imagawa M, Naruse S, Tsuji S, Fujioka A, Yamaguchi H. Coenzyme Q10, iron and vitamin B_6 in genetically-confirmed Alzheimer's disease. *Lancet* 340: 671, 1992.

Conclusion

SUMMARY. The interpretation of chronic fatigue syndrome as a limbic dysfunction in a dysregulated neuroimmune network is reviewed. It is stressed that this model does not preclude several pathophysiologic models, any one of which could be supported by the limbic hypothesis: that is, CFS is a viral syndrome or post-viral syndrome, CFS is an immune dysfunction, CFS is a neurologic disease, or CFS is a metabolic/nutritional/toxic/hypersensitivity disorder. Challenges facing future CFS research are noted, and hope is expressed for a new awareness of CFS as an epidemic which is poorly understood if even acknowledged.

At the present level of understanding it would appear that chronic fatigue syndrome is a limbic encephalopathy. Since it is multicausal, and since limbic function can be modulated in numerous ways, it is most productive to consider diagnosis and treatment in a multiaxial format, as is suggested in DSM-III-R, or in the context of the biopsychosocial model, which views health and disease in a descending hierarchy from the biosphere to subatomic particles. David Levin and George Solomon discuss this model in the context of PNI.[1]

It is not my purpose here to view CFS as a socially-conditioned symptom choice, although it appears that neurasthenic syndromes are more common in societies in which somatic symptoms are more socially sanctioned, and there is a cultural mechanism by which a limbic encephalopathy produced by cognitive (heteromodal and paralimbic) and affective (limbic) alterations could occur.

[DocuSerial™ co-indexing entry]

"Conclusion," Goldstein, J.A. Published in: *Haworth Library of the Medical Neurobiology of Somatic Disorders* (The Haworth Medical Press), Volume 1, 1993 and *Chronic Fatigue Syndromes: The Limbic Hypothesis*, Goldstein, J.A., The Haworth Medical Press, 1993.

189

Nor do I wish to look at CFS particularly as a result of disintegration and pollution of the biosphere, with thinning of the ozone layer, poisoning of the food chain, toxic waste dumps, and hazards of electromagnetic radiation. These issues may be germane to CFS in the context of clinical ecology, but are difficult to quantitate and are generally beyond the purview of this book.

Viewing CFS as a response to impaired interpersonal relations at home or in the workplace is a little more germane to the production of stress and avoidant techniques that may alter limbic functioning, but are addressed in the context of the limbic hypothesis primarily from the standpoint of cognitive-behavioral therapy. Whether the 1980s and 1990s are more stressful than other historical eras is open for discussion.

There remain five types of pathophysiology that should be considered. They are not independent of one another, and all five could conceivably interact in a single patient:

1. *CFS is a viral or post-viral syndrome.* A persistent viral infection of lymphocytes and/or neurons could alter cell function in CFS and cause the panoply of symptoms, signs, laboratory/neuropsychological/imaging abnormalities that have been reported. This etiology was addressed by many researchers early in the history of CFS and is still maintained by some. A corollary hypothesis is that a virus is no longer present, but that enduring derangements of cellular function exist, predominantly in the production of various transmitter substances which could cause neurologic and immune dysfunction. A second corollary is that a viral antigen displayed on the surface of an infected cell could cause an autoimmune disorder and that CFS is one such disease. A third corollary is that a CFS retrovirus could encode a superantigen which could cause autoimmune disorders by activating T-cell receptors. An absence of inflammatory cells in CFS biopsy specimens argues against this hypothesis. A fourth corollary would be that cytokines could be one of the neurotoxic gene products encoded by a CFS retrovirus. A fifth corollary could be that T-cell activation is secondary to another virus, such as HHV-6, that may proliferate as a result of CFS immunosuppression.

2. *CFS is an immune dysfunction.* In this scenario, CFS is viewed primarily as a disorder of immune activation, perhaps a distinctive kind of immune activation, possibly with a definable failure of suppressor T-cell function. The pathophysiology of such a disease would be the generation of inappropriate types and amounts of cytokines, but the etiology of the immune dysfunction is perceived to be indeterminate, or of secondary importance to the dysregulation of physiology wreaked by the cytokines. This abnormal production of cytokines could not just be a result of various infections, but also of genetic alterations in processing, presentation, or generation of cytokine mRNA, as well as in deranged cytokine receptor regulation and production of second (and third) messengers. Since there is bidirectional communication between the immune and nervous systems, a primary immune dysfunction could result in a psychoneuroimmunologic disorder, perhaps with various immunotransmitter "codes" as proposed by Besedovsky. There are also immunoactive cells in the brain which could initiate the process. A good argument for CFS being a viral and/or immune dysfunction is the efficacy of Ampligen, an antiviral and immunomodulatory compound that has a highly specific (as far as is now known) pharmacologic effect on one antiviral enzyme system. There is no other drug used in humans that has this mode of action. Ampligen has no intrinsic mood-altering properties. It has not been tested to see whether it can attenuate opioid withdrawal. It has potent effects on the cognitive and affective components of CFS. Cytokines have been demonstrated to have marked CNS effects, and receptors for IL-1 are dense primarily in limbic areas and in the choroid plexus. It is possible that immune activation markers may be epiphenomena in many CFS patients. The role of IL-1 as a stress cytokine is pivotal in causing many CFS CNS symptoms. IL-1 mRNA is found in the anterior temporal lobe and we consistently find right anterior temporal hypoperfusion in our depressed and non-depressed CFS patients. IL-1 can be released by stress, infection, or immune dysfunction. IL-1 beta, which can act at a distance, would be more likely to play a role in CFS than IL-1 alpha, which acts locally. Central IL-1 beta causes CRH-mediated immunosuppression in shocked rats, whether they are adrenalectomized or not, apparently by neurologic pathways to the peripheral immune system.

3. *CFS is a neurologic disease.* This view is the focus of the book. I would not be as restrictive as one investigator who asked me: "So do you think CFS is a hepatitis of the brain?" although in many cases it probably is, without the inflammatory component. I hope that by now I have demonstrated that postulating a limbic encephalopathy is the most parsimonious mechanism to explain symptom generation, physical signs, and test abnormalities. Fatigue, like pain in CFS, is central, and is doubtless mediated by a neural network. Certain people, in certain situations, may be genetically more predisposed to experience fatigue, perhaps even expressing a certain proto-oncogene like c fos which has been demonstrated in stressed rats. I have been impressed that patients not only with premorbid mood disorders, but also with premorbid bruxism and sleep disorders in the absence of any mood disorder, are more likely to develop CFS. In such patients, a limbic encephalopathy, in a more limited sense, already existed. Our research, as well as that of others, indicates that there is a CNS dysfunction in CFS. One finding that I have previously mentioned supports the idea that limbic dysfunction in CFS patients is pre-cognitive and may not be caused solely by "somatosensory amplification." Twelve CFS patients tested with auditory-evoked response measurement had abnormalities in the P100 component. This epoch occurs as the neural impulse is emerging from the brain stem into the hippocampus and before it would have reached the auditory cortex or the association areas, i.e., before awareness (cognition) of the stimulus could have occurred. Furthermore, if somatosensory amplification were a primary etiologic feature of CFS, I would expect to see abnormalities in somatosensory evoked responses. Hundreds of my patients have had SERs as part of a BEAM scan protocol, and none have been abnormal, although AERs and/or VERs are almost always more than two standard deviations from the mean of the control group, especially in the temporal lobes. Thus I believe that CFS patients have a neurologic disorder that may cause them to have somatosensory amplification, although there is obvious potential for a chicken-egg argument here. A paralimbic dysfunction is one possible candidate. Such a distinction may eventually need to be made, if life experiences (psychiatric) caused a limbic encephalopathy as opposed to, say, viruses (neurologic). A similar disclaimer could be

made for hyperventilation. Does a misperception of ventilatory feedback result in the vicious cycle of hyperventilation → physiologic change → anxiety → more hyperventilation start with the hyperventilation or the anxiety? Our findings of irregular respiratory rhythm during maximal exercise suggest a primary derangement in central respiratory regulation, perhaps in limbic regulation of automatic respiration, as previously discussed. Endorphin hyposecretion could also cause hyperventilation, since opioids suppress respiration. Other examples could be cited, but I do not wish to belabor this point.

It is difficult at this time to know what role to assign neuroendocrine abnormalities in CFS. The alterations in HPA axis function studied in depression for over a decade have not yielded much in the way of therapeutic advances, and augmentation of antidepressant effect with thyroid hormone has yielded only modest results. There may be value in trying to manipulate IGF-1 levels in fibromyalgia patients, since they have been found to have decreased levels of this substance. Efforts to stimulate secretion of CRH, TRH, or GHRH have been therapeutically unrewarding, although the notion that neurasthenic and chronic pain states could be characterized by a deficiency of one or more of these hypothalamic hormones and/or a dysregulation of their secretion by transmitter substances secreted by higher centers is an attractive one.

An impediment to the integration of neuroendocrine findings into the psychoneuroimmunology of CFS is that if IL-1 levels are elevated, CRH levels should be, also. IL-1 also has a direct potentiating effect on the pituitary for the release of proopiomelanocortin (POMC)-derived peptides induced by a variety of secretagogues including CRH. CRH even upregulates IL-1 receptors in mouse AtT-20 pituitary tumor cells, and IL-2 receptors in lymphocytes. I am not able to resolve this paradox except to postulate that in those patients with high IL-1 levels there must also be high levels of IL-1 antagonist to block its effect. If IL-1 levels in CSF are normal, there may be a local dysregulation of IL-1 secretion. If IL-1 secretion is normal, there may be disorders in intermediary substances between IL-1 and CRH such as IL-6, serotonin, or PGF_2-alpha.[2] We are currently testing a hypothesis that elevations in IL-1 levels produced by exercise stimulate the secretion of CRH and ACTH and GH in normals, and that this effect may be blocked in CFS. Preliminary results demonstrate the expected increase in IL-1 post-exercise, but little or no increase in cortisol or growth hormone. Pre-exercise IL-1 levels are normal. These findings suggest a CFS defect in the central action of IL-1.

It would be tempting to treat CFS patients with corticosteroids or ACTH. Some physicians are doing so, and anecdotal reports of success abound. Corticosteroids have effects on the CNS at various sites, and can thus produce a variety of effects. They have numerous mechanisms of action: increasing arousal in the reticular activating system by altering norepinephrine metabolism; direct effects on target cells in the limbic system, especially the hippocampus; increasing norepinephrine uptake of cortical and limbic neurons; reducing CNS serotonin levels by shunting tryptophan away from serotonin and toward kallurenin; altering the sodium-potassium pump, levels of cAMP, cGMP, acetylcholine, dopamine, and beta endorphin.[3]

Corticosteroids can cause mild euphoria and diminished fatigue in certain individuals; this effect is dose-related. Pre-existing psychiatric history has no relationship to developing steroid-induced mood disorders, including psychosis, but steroid euphoria has been related to abuse of this substance. Steroid treatment of CFS should be attempted with caution. Researchers are beginning to target modulation of symptoms caused by neural effects of cytokines such as IL-1. These symptoms are called "sickness behavior,"[4] and are manifested in experimental animals by passivity and reduced exploration.

4. *CFS is a psychiatric disorder.* Patients with temporolimbic epilepsy sometimes have bizarre sensations, experiences, and behaviors. It can be difficult to know "what is the epilepsy and what is me?" Whether "mind" or "consciousness" is a product of brain function at a certain degree of complexity has long been debated. In a sense, all cases of CFS could be psychiatric disorders, if psychiatry became behavioral neurology. Viewing psychiatric disorders in general as limbic pathophysiology would accelerate a gradually developing tendency toward consideration of functional neuroanatomic principles and broaden the purview of the discipline. Psychia-

trists would then have to be knowledgeable in limbic physiology, all systems regulated by the limbic system, and all systems which regulate the limbic system. Disorders of these systems and their treatments would have to be part of the knowledge base, which would be increasingly shared by many other medical specialties.

Besides incorporating the idea of the limbic system as the master regulator of the brain and body, the other revolutionary impact that CFS will have on psychiatry is that viral infection can fairly commonly produce behavioral morbidity which may be long-lasting. Whether or not one currently believes that CFS may be caused by a virus, there is agreement that neurobehavioral abnormalities seen in AIDS are probably due to persistent HIV infection causing cells to function abnormally. They may produce toxic substances such as EAAs, gp120, and gp160, or inappropriate amounts of cytokines. As previously discussed, gp120 may block the effect of VIP on neurons, and peptide T, as a VIP agonist, may ameliorate this effect. It is possible that gp120 may have a similar role in causing HIV-induced CD4 depletion, and could explain how so few HIV-infected cells could produce such disastrous consequences. An effect of the VIP antagonism may be decreased production of a newly described growth factor which may be involved in the CD4 lymphopenia.[5] Reverse transcriptase inhibitors and protease inhibitors may have some effect on this process; AIDS dementia is less common since zidovudine has been prescribed earlier in the course of the illness. Using HIV "tat" gene inhibitors may be a more promising approach.[6] The HIV tat gene produces a protein which greatly increases the activity of the virus. Without tat, the virus becomes inactive. Tat gene inhibitors would be effective in chronically infected cells, and it appears that HIV does not develop resistance to these agents. Treating "psychiatric" disorders with antiviral drugs would be at least as profound an advance as the introduction of neuroleptic and antidepressant agents. The primary benefit of research by non-psychiatric physicians in CFS, who considered it to be a purely "organic" disease, may be to advance the use of antiviral and immunomodulatory agents (such as Ampligen) in psychiatry by a decade or more.

The CNS ramifications of AIDs have recently been summarized.[7] The findings parallel much of what is discussed in this book.

5. *CFS is a metabolic/nutritional/toxic/hypersensitivity/disorder.*
It appears that certain patients have their illness triggered by potentially toxic substances. Encephalopathies with distinctive neuropsychological test and PET scan results have been best described in patients with organophosphate insecticide exposure, but tung oil and hydrocarbons are also likely candidates. Heavy metal poisoning and carbon monoxide intoxication on a chronic basis should be considered. "Sick building syndrome" is a real entity.

Patients with environmental allergy, multiple chemical sensitivity, and "brain allergy" may have a limbic encephalopathy, and the finding that there is a high premorbid incidence of mood disorders in this population would further predispose them to a more extensive degree of limbic dysfunction. Food intolerance in this group could be a result of deranged release of transmitter substances postprandially, improper digestion of foods to release exogenous benzodiazepines or opioids ("exorphins"), abnormal limbic receptors for such substances (my choice), or release of metabolites as has been proposed for candida. Persistent GI infection with yeast, giardia, or other microorganisms could derange gastrointestinal physiology, as could viral infections of the myenteric plexus.[8] These various factors could act alone or in combination.

Since we are only a few thousand years from the hunter-gatherer stage, it may be that we are still nutritionally adapted to that level of sustenance. Patients on macrobiotic diets can reverse atherosclerosis, and a recent report attested to the efficacy of a vegetarian diet in treating rheumatoid arthritis.[9] Many sorts of relative metabolic blocks could be postulated in CFS, and nutritional strategies abound for dealing with them. I have not had much success with this approach, but I probably have a sampling bias in my patient population. Even nutritional approaches addressed to neurochemical interventions, such as low-tyramine diets, are only mildly helpful (with the notable exception of alcohol avoidance).

If CFS patients had a mitochondrial defect, most often seen in myopathies and severe hereditary neurologic dysfunction, strategies to intervene at this level, other than nutritionally, could be devised.

It may be that CFS patients could be divided into four categories, which may be sub-typed into responders and non-responders to nitroglycerin:

1. Those with acute viral onset who meet the new diagnostic criteria very strictly.
2. Those who do not quite meet the criteria and/or may not have an acute viral onset.
3. Those with concomitant medical problems.
4. Those with concomitant, or pre-existing psychiatric problems which are not just reactive to having a chronic illness.

I would hypothesize that group 1 would be most apt to be viral culture positive, and most likely to respond to antiviral chemotherapy as the primary treatment. An antiviral agent would have to pass the blood-brain barrier to treat a virally-induced limbic encephalopathy. All groups would require a multi-modal diagnostic and treatment approach, but with varying degrees of emphasis, depending on the etiologic factors. An environment modeled on a chronic pain unit, where antimicrobial, immunomodulatory, and neuropharmacologic agents were available, could help recalcitrant cases. Outpatient treatment with a component of cognitive-behavioral therapy would be appropriate for most patients. Programs should be able to provide cognitive retraining, functional capacity evaluations, work hardening, and gradual conditioning. Those suitable for more rapid conditioning with reattribution could possibly be identified by brain SPECT.

The finding of limbic/prefrontal abnormalities in all CFS patients augments the distinction between CFS and depression, and between "physical" and "mental," and lends support to a certain type of somatization as relevant to CFS physiology. The fact that CFS patients have a specific localization of prefrontal hypoperfusion lends more evidence to the assertion that CFS is not depression, but may be more productively viewed as a limbic encephalopathy, with IL-1 beta and CRH as the predominant neuroimmune transmitters involved, and with anterior temporal lobe dysfunction being a unifying characteristic. There are probably multiple central IL-1 beta receptors and antagonists, and many neuroregulatory substances that attenuate and potentiate its effects.[10] PET scan results are similar to SPECT and distinguish CFS patients from those with major depression, normal controls, and AIDS.

It is possible to offer a hypothetical mechanism of action for production of CFS symptoms. My thinking, as that of others, has centered around "the idea of a universal system of peptide-mediated molecular events that serve to fine-tune function within the cells that compose many of the body's complex regulatory networks."[11] Such a synthesis has recently been attempted by Chrousos and Gold[12] who offer "a new perspective on human disease states associated with dysregulation of the stress system." Their model involves hyper- or hypofunction of the CRH/locus ceruleus-norepinephrine autonomic nervous systems and "their peripheral effectors, the pituitary-adrenal axis, and the limbs of the autonomic nervous system." Most of the information discussed in their article deals with neuroregulators, but possible viral modulation of them is not mentioned and regulation of such systems by paralimbic and heteromodal areas is scarcely discussed. The authors did not have the benefit of the functional neuroimaging or neuropsychologic data previously mentioned. Viewing IL-1 as a more central regulator of the functions they discuss explains CFS symptomatology more completely.

A comprehensive hypothesis should account for why CFS is made worse by stress, exercise, infection, and possibly nasal allergy. The first three stimuli release IL-1 alpha, which is membrane bound and acts locally, and IL-1 beta, which can act distantly in the manner of a neuropeptide.[13] Ampligen decreased serum levels of IL-1 alpha in responders; IL-1 beta was not measured. Almost nothing is known about the effect of Ampligen in the brain. Poly I: Poly C, a related compound with a longer duration of action, has a central action since its effects on the immune system can be conditioned,[14] but no one has investigated this mechanism. Poly I: Poly C increases levels of IL-1 in the periphery. If it also does so in the brain, an effect of Ampligen might be to increase production of central IL-1 beta, thus overcoming inhibition of its effect.

Besides retrograde transport of neuropeptides from the nasal mucosa, other mechanisms of the influence of nasal allergy on central IL-1 beta secretion include the fact that histamine stimulates the increased production of IL-1 beta by cells that secrete it via the H-2 receptor,[15] but suppresses TNF-alpha by the same mechanism.[16] Such findings may account for the benefit sometimes seen in CFS when H-2 receptor antagonists are prescribed. IL-1 beta has been detected in the rat olfactory tubercle[17] and could be released in patients with nasal allergy as well as those with environmental sensitivities. Dysregulation of olfaction could occur if IL-1 beta action is inhibited or stimulated.

IL-1 beta increases the secretion of somatostatin, growth hormone, and TSH. Somatostatin, which is also induced by CRH, decreases secretion of GH and thus somatomedin-C. When we have measured post-exercise somatostatin levels in our patients, they have been low. Somatomedin-C (IGF-1) has been reported to be decreased in fibromyalgia, but probably not by hypersecretion of CRH. One might wonder whether those who manifest somatosensory amplification have an altered IL-1 beta receptor status in certain paralimbic or heteromodal neurons which may exhibit decreased dendritic synaptogenesis as the mechanism of maladaptive augmented informational transfer. This situation could be modified by cognitive-behavioral therapy.

It has been speculated that levels of IL-1ra may be major modulators of IL-1 activity and that IVIG may increase IL-1ra levels.[18] Certain patients appear to respond to IVIG, although the reason why they do so is still obscure. There was a trend to increase peripheral IL-1ra levels in our CFS patients post-exercise. IL-6 was never detected.

Transforming growth factor-beta downregulates the binding of labeled IL-1 to T-cells and bone marrow cells.[19] Since peripheral blood mononuclear lymphocytes (PBMLs) of CFS patients secrete increased quantities of TGF-beta, it is possible that similar altered regulation occurs in the brain.

If a retrovirus is a candidate for producing CFS symptoms centrally, a neurotoxic gene product should be involved. The retroviral envelope protein p15E, a 17-amino acid peptide derived from the envelope protein of T-lymphotropic retroviruses, blocks IL-1 mediated signal transduction, but does not interfere with the IL-1 receptor or the IL-1 molecule itself.[20] Transactivating viruses such as HHV-6, by increasing retroviral activity, should increase the production of such proteins. Ampligen could treat CFS by inhibiting HHV-6 and/or a retrovirus.

Some of the CNS effects of IL-1 beta are mediated through IL-6 and/or serotonin. Fluoxetine and MAOIs increase serotonin levels by different mechanisms and are effective in CFS. Ritanserin, a $5HT_{1c}/5HT_2$ receptor antagonist, markedly improved pain and fatigue in an open study of fibromyalgia patients which I performed. Some patients had a marked worsening of symptoms, often to degrees of severity they had not previously experienced, when ritanserin was discontinued. Such an effect of ritanserin discontinuation has not been observed in other patient groups, but a similar response was noted in Ampligen patients when the experiment was terminated. Ritanserin appears to have efficacy in opioid, and possibly cocaine withdrawal,[21] and if it was able to increase CRH biosynthesis, then the secretion of endogenous opioids and catecholamines may have been increased as well. The localization of the $5HT_{1c}$ receptor is similar to areas where IL-1 beta is synthesized. I have noted that some CFS patients are dramatically improved by small doses of an opioid (e.g., half of a Darvocet) for 1-3 days. This response suggests upregulation of mu receptors, possibly due to a beta endorphin deficiency.

Ondansetron, a $5HT_3$ receptor antagonist, blocks the pyrogenic effects of IL-1 beta. Since IL-1 can also cause gastric stasis as a central effect,[22] it may also produce nausea by a similar mechanism. Pre- and post-treatment cortisols in CFS patients with intractable nausea who have received ondansetron do not change. As previously noted, fenfluramine, a 5HT agonist, has not benefitted my patients.

PGE_2 and PGF_2 may be intermediaries in the effects of IL-1 alpha and IL-1 beta, respectively. Provision of exogenous essential fatty acids could increase these eicosanoids, while viral infections, perhaps by inhibiting delta-6 desaturase, the enzyme which converts linoleic to gamma linoleic acid, could decrease them.

Augmenting the synthesis and release of CRH in CFS would make sense, but appears difficult to accomplish. Fenfluramine, reported to be an effective secretagogue in other situations,[23] is ineffective, as is DDAVP.[24] An agent worth trying would be a thymic peptide such as thymopentin or alpha-1 thymosin which appears to increase CRH secretion,[25] or perhaps only ACTH, by a direct mechanism. Protein kinase C stimulates CRH production, and CFS/FM lymphocytes are deficient in this kinase where stimulated with IL-2. Low doses of phorbol esters may be of benefit, although high doses may be harmful. Research on the neuroendocrine thymus gives conflicting results. One study finds CRH in rat thymus,[26] while another reports that intraventricular thymosin alpha-1 decreases ACTH and TSH but stimulates it when given at the pituitary level.[27]

It is difficult to explain the action of antidepressants in CFS by an effect on CRH-sympathetic interaction, since all classes of antidepressants appear to attenuate CRH effect on the locus ceruleus.[28] A direct modulatory effect on the SNS or on hippocampal glucocorticoid receptors is more likely. No research has been done on the effects of antidepressants on IL-1. Decreased blood flow to muscle and brain could be a result of a dysautonomic process, and muscle perfusion abnormalities have been reported in fibromyalgia. Excitatory amino acids release IL-1 and both substances have been implicated in neuronal injury, especially in neurodegenerative conditions. Mice infected with lymphocytic choriomeningitis (LCM) virus have characteristic problems with learning which are worsened by scopolamine challenge.[29] IL-1 levels in the CNS have not been measured in this model. Since acetylcholine also induces CRH release, it would be interesting to try tacrine (Cognex), a cholinesterase inhibitor, in the cognitively impaired CFS patient with persistent viral infection. Such patients should also have a positive scopolamine challenge test, used to diagnose patients with Alzheimer's disease. If some of the same neuroregulatory substances are involved in CFS patients without apparent viral infection, tacrine should still be potentially useful, assuming that findings in LCM mice can be generalized to humans with CFS. Cytokines such as IL-6, TNF-alpha, TGF-beta, and interferons are all released in chronic CNS viral infections, although from astrocytes and glial cells, rather than from neurons. The same cytokine cascade as that induced by viruses occurs in transgenic mice who have had the IL-6 gene inserted.[30]

IL-1 dysregulation could also be implicated in anxiety, since the cytokine augments the effects of GABA at the $GABA_A$ receptor by increasing GABA-mediated increase in chloride conductance.[31] IL-1 alone has no effect on chloride conductance. GABA has an inhibitory effect on the CRH and sympathetic nervous systems (along with dynorphin).[32]

IL-1 effects occur at various concentrations in the brain, from nanogram to femtogram amounts. Most of the functions involved in CFS require very low IL-1 levels, more evidence for impaired signal transduction or a receptor disorder as being a likely mechanism.

Although a dysregulation of hippocampal IL-1 beta action producing a limbic encephalopathy with multiple etiologic determinants is an attractive hypothesis, the situation is undoubtedly more complicated than this and awaits further unraveling of the mystery. A small minority of patients we have tested have a relatively normal neuroendocrine response to exercise yet have the characteristic worsening of symptoms. A more complete evaluation of this process may involve placement of a lumbar subarachnoid catheter for a more direct assessment of regulatory substances.

It is possible to conceive of a functional neuroanatomic model for CFS at this point, assigning a central role to the hippocampus, perhaps even to the dentate gyrus. Selective neurochemical destruction by colchicine of one link in the intrinsic hippocampal circuitry, the dentate gyrus granule cells and their mossy fiber axons, caused a dramatic decrease in CRH expression in the paraventricular nucleus.[33]

Dentate gyrus cells innervate hippocampal fields in a multisynaptic fashion, with glutamate appearing to be the transmitter released at cell synapses. Colchicine destroys excitatory glutamatergic synapses, leaving GABAergic inhibitory synapses intact.

Since cells that secrete IL-1 may be co-localized with glutamatergic neurons, a multifactorial functional abnormality of dentate gyrus cells could be involved in CFS. The activity of the dorsolateral prefrontal cortex could be altered by modulation of the well-known pathway from the hippocampus → fornix → mammillary body → mammillothalamic tract → anterior thalamus → prefrontal cortex → paralimbic areas, especially insula and cingulate gyrus → hippocampus.

There are three groups of glutamate receptors:

1. N-methyl-D aspartate (NMDA),
2. alpha-amino-3-hydroxy-5-methyl-4-isoxazolepropionate (AMPA)-Kainate, and
3. metabotropic receptors.

Receptor subtypes exist in each group and appear to have different localizations and functions: mRNA for the $NMDAR_2$ subunit has been localized by in situ hybridization in rat brain. There are four subtypes of $NMDAR_2$, all of which can be co-expressed with the seven types of $NMDAR_1$ receptor, allowing for considerable functional heterogeneity.[34] The subtype (in the rat) which may be most relevant to CFS is the $NMDAR_{2A}$, which is prominently expressed in the hippocampus and cerebral cortex. Developing agonists for these receptors may enable us to treat CFS and related disorders more effectively.

Invoking a glutamatergic mechanism could explain the sudden, epileptoid changes in function experienced by CFS patients and could transduce behavioral state variables and alterations in neuroelectrical function into neurochemical modification. A perturbation in this circuit in the hippocampal, prefrontal, or paralimbic areas, as a result of exercise, stress, infection, hypoxia, cognitive activity, sleep deprivation, or any of the numerous other CFS precipitants, could cause the diverse, yet familiar, symptomatology which patients experience. Different transmitter substances are present in different regions, and variability in presentation could be determined by the region most affected. Alterations in the function of G proteins may be involved in rapid state changes,[35] and may serve an integrative function in neural networks.

Understanding the relationship of multiple CNS cytokines with other neuroregulators, neurotoxic gene products, possible endogenous viral analogs such as dsRNA, second and third messengers, EAAs, nitric oxide, G proteins, 2,5A, proto-oncogenes, and possibly superantigens is a daunting challenge, but one which is being undertaken.

I am doing so in collaboration with members of the exercise ergometry laboratory at Harbor-UCLA Medical Center. CFS patients undergo maximum exercise by bicycle ergometry. [133]Xenon brain SPECT scans, core body temperature measurement, and blood drawn by venipuncture are done before and after exercise. Various physiologic parameters are measured during exercise. Another [133]Xenon brain SPECT scan is performed the next day. Exercise was chosen as a stimulus to assess the functional changes seen in CFS since its intensity and effects can be precisely measured in the setting of a physiologic laboratory. Other stressors such as slow-wave sleep deprivation, cognitive tasks, viral infections, or testing "on a bad day" could have also been chosen but would have been more difficult to implement.

A model of peripheral and/or central interferences with IL-1 beta action in CFS would predict, among other things[36], that after exercise, as distinct from normals:

1. cortisol response would be blunted,[37]
2. growth hormone would be blunted,[38]
3. catecholamine response would be blunted,[39]
4. endorphins would not increase as much as in normals,[40, 41], and enhancement of dopamine release by stimulation of mu-2 receptors in the mesocortical and mesolimbic dopaminergic projections would be decreased,[42]
5. IL-1 would increase[43,44] but IL-6 would not,[45]
6. temperature would not increase as much as in normals, and might even decrease,[46]
7. regional cerebral blood flow would decrease if IL-1 beta is involved in maintaining cerebral vasodilatation[47] and since IL-1ra mRNA is found in cerebral vessels.[48]

Although the testing process continues as of this writing, all predictions have been fulfilled, quite to the consternation of the physicians in the exercise laboratory. Some patients demonstrate a very rapid hyperventilation at the onset of exercise, a phenomenon not previously observed, but reported when exercising subjects were given naloxone.[49] We have previously discussed how the limbic system mediates automatic respiration. Beta-endorphin levels may be one of the neuroregulators involved in the deranged functional neuroanatomy of CFS/FM.

IL-1 beta leads to induction of nitric oxide synthase which synthesizes nitric oxide (NO) from L-arginine with tetrahydrobiopterin (BH4), flavin adenine dinucleotide (FAD), and flavin mononucleotide (FMN) as necessary co-factors. NO is released continuously in varying amounts to regulate blood vessel tone as a vasodilator. Local changes in expression of NO synthase may be produced by alterations in the balance of cytokines such as IL-1, which induce

NO synthase, and those such as TGF-beta[50] and IL-10[51] which inhibit induction. Such inhibitory factors may be involved in the decrease in regional cerebral blood flow which we usually observe in CFS patients after exercise. NO is also thought to be a mediator of slow synaptic transmission and is thought to be important in memory and learning processes. IL-10 has a high homology to a product of EBV called BCRF-1[52] and it has been speculated that EBV has appropriated this gene from the human genome. IL-10 inhibits the synthesis of cytokines by TH1 cells, a member of a pair of mutually inhibitory subsets of T-cells. TH1 cells inhibit TH2 cells, which produce IL-4 and IL-5 which lead to some of the major manifestations of allergy. IL-10 production may bias an immune response towards allergy.[53]

If inhibition of NO synthase is involved in the pathophysiology of CFS/FM, it should be possible to bypass this block by supplying exogenous NO. A safe and rapidly effective way to augment NO levels is by administering nitroglycerin and then longer-acting nitrates if the nitroglycerin is effective.

As of this writing I have treated sixty CFS patients with 0.04-0.15 mg of sublingual nitroglycerin. Higher doses are not usually effective. Forty-four of these patients met criteria for fibromyalgia with 11/18 tender points. Thirty-one of the patients had a beneficial response, and most of the responders also had fibromyalgia. Responders often reported feeling very relaxed, almost euphoric. Usually their pain was decreased. Many had more energy, and some reported amelioration of "brain fog." These gains seemed to be maintained with very low doses of longer-acting nitrates. Formal experiments are being planned. Even if nitroglycerin does not prove to be an effective long-term therapeutic agent, it may still be useful as a pharmacologic probe.

Some patients, however, develop rapid tolerance to the effects of nitroglycerin. Nitroglycerin rarely makes anyone worse, but there is experimental evidence to suggest that one cannot merely "dump" nitric oxide into a neuronal network. When studied in the CA1 region of rat hippocampal slices, nitric oxide was found to "play a positive or negative modulatory role in long-term potentiation depending on prior events at the tetanized synapse and the ambient concentration of excitatory amino acids."[54] The modulation of synaptic transmission is quite precise. It might be possible to increase nitric oxide synthesis more physiologically by administering its precursor, arginine, or a co-factor for nitric oxide synthesis, such as tetrahydrobiopterin. But "the intracellular levels of arginine are already high and the supply of arginine is not normally rate-limiting for the constitutive enzyme. Whether the situation differs in disease states associated with reduced synthesis of nitric oxide remains to be determined."[55]

Most CFS patients who do not have a beneficial response to low dose nitroglycerin nevertheless experience unusual reactions. They can feel intoxicated, dysphoric, or depressed, or extremely agitated ("like I've had twelve cups of coffee"). Two individuals have stated that they feel like they inhaled nitrous oxide (N_2O), not usually thought to be a product of nitroglycerin. An occasional patient will have no response at all, even to a 0.6 mg dose. A few patients have not responded until such high levels have been reached. In an apparent non-responder to nitroglycerin, I administer consecutive low sub-lingual doses until symptoms of nitroglycerin effect, such as headache or lightheadedness, occur, signifying the endpoint of dosage titration. Some patients may not respond immediately to nitroglycerin, but respond to low doses of long-acting agents after about two weeks. Patients who have worsening symptomatology after taking nitroglycerin may respond to niacinamide, 500 mg TID, in about two weeks, Niacinamide may function as a partial NO antagonist. Another partial NO antagonist, atropine, does not improve these patients. Tolerance to the therapeutic effect has been a problem. In angina, tolerance to nitroglycerin is related to low levels of cyclic GMP. It can be modified by intermittent dosing, or strategies to enhance the conversion of nitroglycerin to nitric oxide could be employed.[56] Trials of methionine and N-acetylcysteine, which have been suggested to stimulate this transformation, have not been effective in CFS. It may be possible to alter the activity of guanylyl cyclase, to increase levels of cyclic GMP, and to enhance the activity of calmodulin or of the specific protein kinases that are stimulated. Guanylyl cyclase can also be activated by carbon monoxide, the hydroxyl radical,[57] and atrial natrurietic factor.[58] Experimental nitrates exist to which tolerance does not seem to develop.

NO synthase can also be stimulated by cholinergic agonists. The best one available clinically is nicotine. I have used a transdermal nicotine patch which can be cut with a scissors without losing nicotine from a reservoir (Nicotrol, Parke-Davis). The lowest potency patch is 5 mg, and one-half a patch usually is sufficient. I have had success with it both in patients who develop nitroglycerin tolerance and in a few who have not responded to nitroglycerin at all. Improvement occurs primarily in levels of energy and alertness, and takes place in about one hour.

Nicotine may exert its effect in CFS by increasing dopamine secretion from cell bodies in the A10 dopaminergic neurons in the ventral tegmentum,[59] which project to the nucleus accumbens in the limbic striatum, and to the prefrontal cortex. The A10 cells are controlled by a specific set of genes,[60] and destroying them causes cognitive disorders and problems in attention.[61] Patients with a history of major depression often get much more depressed when they stop smoking.[62] Smoking reduces levels of Parkinsonism in schizophrenic patients taking neuroleptics.[63] Even though 2.5 mg of nicotine per day is a very low dose, a risk/benefit analysis should be done with the CFS patient before prescribing it. Those with a history of drug dependence should be monitored very closely. Tolerance may not develop to this nicotine dose, since the sub-group of A10 neurons that projects to the dorsolateral prefrontal cortex lacks autoreceptors.[64]

A possible mechanism of the analgesia induced by nitroglycerin may have to do with stress-induced analgesia, which is classified as "opioid" and "non-opioid," depending on whether it is antagonized by naloxone or not. Opioids are not particularly effective in fibromyalgia. Non-opioid stress-induced analgesia may be blocked by the NMDA receptor antagonist MK-801[65] suggesting that glutamatergic transmission may be impaired in fibromyalgia. NO analgesia has not been blocked in a rat model using MK-801, however.[66]

Malic acid has been advocated as a treatment for fibromyalgia.[67] Nitric oxide synthase has been identified as NADPH-diaphorase. Malic acid is involved in the function of an enzyme which converts NADP into NADPH, used as a substrate for NADPH-diaphorase,[68] and exogenous malic acid may work by enhancing nitric oxide synthase levels, even if sufficient IL-1 beta is not present.

We have measured serum IL-1ra before and after exercise. There is a trend for IL-1ra to increase. IL-1ra, as well as other IL-1 inhibitors, could increase when IL-1 beta does not.[69] We are also measuring somatostatin levels since the failure of growth hormone to increase is our most reliable finding. Somatostatin secretion is regulated in numerous ways, but is increased by IL-1 beta and CRH. Somatostatin levels tend to be low in CFS patients post-exercise.

Since IL-1 beta also induces the secretion of serotonin in the brain,[70] there should be low levels of CSF 5-HIAA in CFS/FM patients. Such a result has been reported,[71] (although another group has found normal levels of CFS biogenic amines in CFS)[72] and is consistent with an interference with central IL-1 beta action at the brain stem dorsal raphe, a region densely populated with serotoninergic neurons, where a high concentration of IL-1 receptor antagonist mRNA has been detected.[73] Levels of dopamine and norepinephrine metabolites are also decreased in the CSF of CFS/FM patients. CSF substance P is increased in FM,[74] and IL-1 beta has been reported to increase substance P levels via the induction of nerve growth factor.[75] Perhaps this pathway is not antagonized.

CSF IL-1 beta is normal in CFS, although alpha interferon may be elevated.[76] Such findings are further evidence that receptor or post-receptor events may be impaired. Alpha and beta interferon induce 2′,5′ oligoadenylate synthetase, especially in the presence of ethanol.[77] Levels of 2,5A have not been measured in the CSF of patients in the Ampligen study, but ethanol could conceivably increase already elevated CNS interferon levels to cause CFS symptoms. Effects of ethanol on other cytokines has not been studied. Interferon has been suggested to augment IgG-induced IL-1ra production,[78] and central alpha interferon can inhibit CRH and stimulate 5HT, as well as shunt tryptophan into the kynurenine pathway. It is difficult, however, to explain all CFS symptoms solely by the effects of elevated central alpha interferon.

TGF-beta concentrations are increased by IL-1[79] and TGF-beta decreases IL-1 receptor expression.[80] The serum level of TGF-beta is increased in CFS,[81] although its alteration by exercise has not been studied. The lipopolysaccharide (LPS)-stimulated release of TGF-beta in peripheral blood mononuclear cell (PBMC) cultures of patients with CFS is suppressed; however, their release of IL-1 beta,

IL-6, and TNF-alpha is increased compared to controls. If LPS stimulation of PBMC is comparable to exercise, the result of increased IL-6 is not consistent with the failure to increase IL-6 that we see in our CFS patients. If exercise increases TGF-beta 1 secretion, then IL-1 beta function could be impaired by receptor downregulation. TGF-beta 1 may increase levels of 2,5A.[82] Although it is generally assumed that 2,5A mRNA must be activated by viral dsRNA in order to transcribe the enzyme,[83] such is not necessarily the case[84,85]; 2,5A may be constitutively expressed in certain disease states. Nuclear RNA from non-infected cells with altered function may also stimulate the enzymes.[86] IL-2 may elevate 2,5A secretion, perhaps mediated by gamma interferon.[87] IL-1 beta effect on 2,5A secretion has not been reported, but TNF alone has no effect.[88] TNF and gamma interferon may have a synergistic effect on 2,5A secretion, however.[89]

Thus, the evidence for interference with the central actions of IL-1 beta in CFS/FM is good. The relationship with 2,5A and EAAs remains to be explored. These substances are more difficult to pharmacologically probe in human subjects with agents that are currently available. Both could be measured in CSF. Patients with AIDS dementia have high levels of CSF quinolinic acid, an EAA.[90] CFS, as well as its many related disorders, may be viewed as a limbic dysregulation of the balance between central IL-1 beta and its numerous endogenous and multifactorially induced exogenous (viral, toxic, environmental) inhibitors. Although the neurochemical pathophysiology is extraordinarily complex, this model provides a basis for rational hypothesis testing and for selecting agents for potential remediation.

Whether my speculations about the possible centrol role of IL-1 beta prove to be true or not, it seems obvious that the integrative function of the limbic system is deranged in CFS and related disorders. One such example is lactate-induced panic. Lactate infusion was not found to increase central lactate or carbon dioxide levels in nonhuman primates. The authors state: "lactate infusion produces peripheral somatic sensations analogous to naturally occurring panic attacks, which the subject then interprets as an indication of an impending internal catastrophe."[91]

One can view the limbic neural network functioning as a computer, processing intero- and exteroceptive stimuli (input), primarily via a bewildering array of chemically transduced messages, integrating them with experiences and attitudes, and selecting responses (output) that should maximize the survival capabilities of the individual.

The limbic system is the highest-order functional regulator in the body, and has effects on fatigue, pain, sleep, weight, appetite, libido, respiration, temperature, blood pressure, memory, attention, concept formation, mood, vigilance, immune and endocrine systems, and the modulation of the peripheral nervous system (to name but a few). If there is limbic dysregulation, any or all of these functions could be deranged.

Such a complex regulatory system could have many specific areas of vulnerability. Dysfunction could have a primary central etiology, or could occur in response to peripheral stressors of various sorts. Since the limbic system is involved in selecting adaptive responses to stress, and stress could be defined as any event which would alter homeostasis, the range of stimuli which could cause limbic dysregulation is large.

Not only might the so-called "functional" disorders be involved, but numerous immunoregulatory diseases could be associated with limbic encephalopathy. Esther Sternberg's CRH-deficient Lewis rats which develop rheumatoid arthritis and behavioral abnormalities are obvious examples, but many conditions associated with immune activation, such as systemic lupus erythematosus or multiple sclerosis, may be implicated. It is common in a CFS practice to see such "overlap" syndromes. Immunosuppression may also be encountered, and some cases of "HIV-negative AIDS" with low CD4 counts and characteristic infections have been followed in CFS practices. Detection of associated viruses may be causes or effects of this immune dysregulation.

The neural network which may be dysfunctional in CFS is similar to that described by Patricia Goldman-Rakic[92] in regard to what she calls "working memory" (short-term memory), in a delayed-response paradigm. She notes that the prefrontal cortex, especially the dorsolateral prefrontal cortex, has "reciprocal connections with more than a dozen distinct cortical association regions (including the superior parietal cortex), premotor centers, caudate nucleus, superior colliculus and brain stem centers." She also describes a circuit between the hippocampus and the prefrontal cortex relating to working memory which appears to be involved in encoding. This circuit may be the same one that we are seeing perturbed in SPECT scans and PET scans. All of the hypometabolic regions (except the anterior cerebellum) seen on PET scans in our CFS patients are in these prefrontal projection areas.

The neural circuitry of obsessive-compulsive disorder (OCD) is the best understood of the neuropsychiatric syndromes. It must be significant that OCD, as diagnosed by DSM-III-R criteria, is almost never comorbid with CFS although obsessional preoccupation with symptomatology is frequently encountered. A "hyperactive" OCD circuit between the orbitofrontal cortex, the cingulate cortex, and the head of the caudate nucleus has been proposed.[93] There are robust excitatory (glutamatergic) projections from both the orbitofrontal and cingulate cortex to the caudate nucleus and ventral striatum (nucleus accumbens).[94] Since the caudate nucleus has efferent inhibitory projections, hypometabolism of the anterior caudate, as we have seen with PET in CFS and others have reported with SPECT[95,96] might provide a neuroanatomic basis for the somatosensory amplification characteristic of CFS. Glutamatergic hypoactivity in this circuit would be compatible with the CFS limbic hypothesis.

The concept of a neural network mediating hemispheric arousal and visuospatial attention has been discussed for the past 15 years. Bipolar depression may be associated with right-sided dysfunction of this system as determined by brain event-related potentials recorded during audiospatial and temporal discrimination tasks. A smaller N100 to left than right hemifield stimuli suggests that the defect might be mediated by subcortical centers.[97] This system may be involved in CFS, especially since, as mentioned previously, Dr. Sandman found a robust difference in P100 between CFS patients with cognitive dysfunction and controls.

Our post-exercise CFS brain SPECT scans demonstrate a predominantly right hemispheric prefrontal, parietal, and temporal hypoperfusion compared to normals. We may be witnessing a derangement of a neural network involved in numerous aspects of functional regulation. An analogous abnormality has been suggested in the left hemisphere in schizophrenic patients.[98] As knowledge of limbic physiology expands, the physicians of the future should be increasingly able to diagnose and treat disorders that are presently poorly understood and imperfectly managed.

REFERENCES

1. Levin DM, Solomon GF. The discursive formation of the body in the history of medicine. *J Med Philosophy* 15:515-537, 1990.

2. Rothwell NJ. Functions and mechanisms of interleukin-1 in the brain. *Trends Pharmacol Sci* 12(11): 430-436, 1991.

3. Hall RCW. Drug-induced psychoses. *Audio-Digest Psychiatry* 20(20), 1991.

4. Kent S, Bluthe R-M, Kelley KW, Dantzer R. Sickness behavior as a new target for drug development. *Trends Pharmacol Sci* 13(1): 24-29, 1992.

5. McGrail M, et al. Peptide T studies: neurophysiologic results. VII Intl. Conf. AIDS, Florence. Vol. 1: 194 (M.B. 2049), 1991.

6. Hsu M-C, Schutt AD, Holly M, Slice LW, Sherman MI, Richman DD, Potash MJ, Volsky DL. Inhibition of HIV replication in acute and chronic infections in vitro by a Tat antagonist. *Science* 254: 1798-1801, 1991.

7. Pequegnat W, Garrick NA, Stover E. Neuroscience findings in AIDS: a review of the research sponsored by the National Institute of Mental Health. *Prog Neuropsychopharmacol Biol Psychiatry* 16: 145-170, 1992.

8. Rosenbaum M, Susser M. *Solving the Puzzle of Chronic Fatigue Syndrome.* Tacoma: Life Sciences Press, 1991.

9. Kjeldsen-Kragh J, Haughen M, Borchgrevink CF, et al. Controlled trial of fasting and one year vegetarian diet in rheumatoid arthritis. *Lancet* 338: 899-902, 1991.

10. Pequegnat W, Garrick NA, Stover E. Neuroscience Findings in AIDS: a review of the research sponsored by the National Institute of Mental Health. *Prog Neuropsychopharmacol Biol Psychiatry* 16: 145-170, 1992.

11. Cooper JR, Bloom FE, Roth R. *The Biochemical Basis of Neuropharmacology,* sixth edition. New York: Oxford University Press, 1991.

12. Chrousos GP, Gold PW. The concept of stress and stress system disorders: overview of physical and behavioral homeostasis. *JAMA* 267(9): 1244-1252, 1992.

13. Rothwell NJ. Functions and mechanisms of interleukin-1 in the brain. *Trends Pharmacol Sci* 12(11): 430-436,1991.

14. Dyck DG, Greenberg AH. Immunopharmacological tolerance as a conditional response dissecting brain-immune pathways. In: Ader R, Felten DF, Cohen N (eds). *Psychoneuroimmunology,* second edition. San Diego: Academic Press, 1991.

15. Vannier E, Dinarello CA. Interleukin-1 induces interleukin-1.VI. Histamine via the H-2 receptor enhances IL-1 induced IL-1 gene expression and synthesis. *Clin Res* (in press).

16. Dinarello CA. Interleukin-1 and interleukin-1 antagonism. *Blood* 77(8): 1627-1652, 1991.

17. Licinio J, Wong M-L, Gold PW. Localization of interleukin-1 receptor antagonist mRNA in rat brain. *Endocrinology* 129(1): 562-564, 1991.

18. Poutsiaka DD, Clark BD, Vannier E, Dinarello CA. Production of interleukin-1 receptor antagonist and interleukin-1 beta by peripheral blood mononuclear cells is differentially regulated. *Blood* 78(5): 1275-1281, 1991.

19. Dinarello CA. Interleukin-1 and interleukin-1 antagonism. *Blood* 77(8): 1627-1652, 1991.

20. Gottleib RA, Lennarz WJ, Knowles RD, Cianciolo GJ, Dinarello CA, Lachman LB, Kleinerman ES. Synthetic peptide corresponding to a conserved domain of the retroviral protein p15E blocks IL-1-mediated signal transduction. *J Immunol* 142: 4321-4325, 1991.

21. Blum P. Personal communication, 1992.

22. Kent S, Bluthe R-M, Kelley KW, Dantzer R. Sickness behavior as a new target for drug development. *Trends Pharmacol Sci* 13: 24-28, 1992.

23. Grice JE, Jackson J, Renfold PJ, Jackson RV. Adrenocorticotropin hyperresponsiveness in myotonic dystrophy following oral fenfluramine administration. *J Neuroendocrinol* 3(1): 69-73, 1991.

24. Martin JB, Reichlin S. *Clinical Neuroendocrinology,* second edition. Philadelphia: FA Davis, 1987.

25. Hall MRS, O'Grady MP, Farah JM. Thymic hormones and immune function: mediation via neuroendocrine circuits. In: Ader R, Felten DF, Cohen N (eds). *Psychoneuroimmunology,* second edition. San Diego: Academic Press, 1991.

26. Redli E. Immuno-reactive and bioactive cortico-tropin releasing factor in rat thymus. *Neuroendocrinology* 55: 115-118, 1992.

27. Milenkovic L, McCann SM. Effects of thymosin alpha-1 on pituitary hormone release. *Neuroendocrinology* 55: 14-19, 1992.

28. Valentino RJ, Curtis AL. Antidepressant interactions with corticotropin-releasing factor in the noradrenergic locus ceruleus. *Psychopharmacol Bull* 27(3): 263-268, 1991.

29. Koob GF, Ehlers CL, Kupfer DJ. *Animal Models of Depression.* Boston, Birkhauser, 1989.

30. Campbell I. Presented at: Chronic Fatigue Syndrome and the Brain. Bel Air, CA, April 1992.

31. Dinarello CA. Interleukin-1 and interleukin-1 antagonism. *Blood* 77(8): 1627-1652, 1991.

32. Chrousos GP, Gold PW. The concept of stress and stress system disorders: overview of physical and behavioral homeostasis. *JAMA* 267(9): 1244-1252, 1992.

33. Brady LS, Lynn AB, Whitfield HJ, Kim H, Herkenham M. Intrahippocampal colchicine alters hypothalamic corticotropin-releasing hormone and hippocampal steroid receptor mRNA in rat brain. *Neuroendocrinology* 55: 121-133, 1992.

34. Nakanishi S. Molecular diversity of glutamate receptors and implications for brain function. *Science* 258:597-603, 1992.

35. Manji H. G proteins: implications for psychiatry. *Am J Psychiatry* 149(6): 749-760, 1992.

36. Simon HB. Exercise and human immune function. In: Ader R, Felten DF, Cohen N. (eds.). *Psychoneuroimmunology,* second edition, San Diego, Academic Press, 1991.

37. Deschenes MR, Kraener WJ, Maresh CM, Crivello JF. Exercise-induced hormonal changes and their effects on skeletal muscle tissue. *Sports Med* 12(2): 80-93, 1991.

38. Deschenes MR, Kraener WJ, Maresh CM, Crivello JF. Exercise-induced hormonal changes and their effects on skeletal muscle tissue. *Sports Med* 12(2): 80-93, 1991.

39. Deschenes MR, Kraemer WJ, Maresh CM, Crivello JF. Exercise-induced hormonal changes and their effects on skeletal muscle tissue. *Sports Med* 12(2): 80-93, 1991.

40. Harber VJ, Sutton JR. Endorphins and exercise. *Sports Med* 1: 154-171, 1984.

41. Hamner MB, Hitri A. Plasma beta-endorphin levels in post-traumatic stress disorder: a preliminary report on exercise-induced stress. *J Neuropsychiatry Clin Neurosci* 4: 59-63, 1992.

42. Wood PL, Rao TS. Morphine stimulation of mesolimbic and mesocortical but not nigrostriatal dopamine release in the rat as reflected by changes in 3-methosyltyramine levels. *Neuropharmacology* 30(4): 399-401, 1991.

43. Simon HB. Exercise and human immune function. In: Ader R, Felten DF, Cohen N. (eds.). *Psychoneuroimmunology,* second edition, San Diego: Academic Press, 1991.

44. Nieman DC, Nehlsen-Cannarella SL. The effect of acute and chronic exercise on immunoglobulins. *Sports Med* 11(3): 183-201,1991.

45. Rothwell NJ. Functions and mechanisms of interleukin-1 in the brain. *Trends Pharmacol Sci* 12(11): 430-436, 1991.

46. Grossman A, Bouloux P, Price P, Drury P, Lam K, Alberti K, Turner T, Besser GM, Sutton JR. The role of opioid peptides in the hormonal responses to acute exercise in man. *Clinic Sci* 67(5): 483-491, 1984.

47. Dinarello CA. Interleukin-1 and interleukin-1 antagonism. *Blood* 77(8): 1627-1652, 1991.

48. Licinio J, Wong M-L, Gold PW. Localization of interleukin-1 receptor antagonist mRNA in rat brain. *Endocrinology* 129(1): 562-564, 1991.

49. Harber VJ, Sutton JR. Endorphins and exercise. *Sports Med* 1: 154-171, 1984.

50. McCall T, Vallance P. Nitric oxide takes centre-stage with newly defined roles. *Trends Pharmacol Sci* 13: 1-6, 1992.

51. Cunha FQ, Moncada S, Liew FW. Interleukin-10 (IL-10) inhibits the induction of nitric oxide synthase by interferon-gamma in murine macrophages. *Biochem Biophys Res Commun* 182(3): 1155-1159, 1992.

52. Durum SK, Quinn DG, Muegge K. New cytokines and receptors make their debut in San Antonio. *Immunol Today* 12(2): 54-57, 1991.

53. Mosmann TR. Regulation of immune responses by T cells with different cytokine secretion phenotypes: role of a new cytokine, cytokine synthesis inhibitory factor (IL-10). *Int Arch Allergy Apply Immunol* 94(1-4): 110-115, 1991.

54. Izumi Y, Clifford DB, Zorumski CF. Inhibition of long-term potentiation by NMDA-mediated nitric oxide release. *Science* 257: 1273-1276, 1992.

55. McCall T, Vallance P. Nitric oxide takes centre-stage with newly defined roles. *Trends Pharmacol Sci* 13: 1-6, 1992.

56. Elkayam V. Tolerance to organic nitrates: evidence, mechanisms, clinical relevance, and strategies for prevention. *Ann Int Med* 114: 667-677, 1991.

57. Schmidt HH. NO, CO, and OH: endogenous soluble guanylyl cyclase-activating factors. *FEBS Lett* 307(1): 102-107, 1992.

58. de Vente J, Steinbusch HW. On the stimulation of soluble and particulate guanylate cyclase in the rat brain and the involvement of nitric oxide as studied by cGMP immunocytochemistry. *Acta Histochem* 92(1): 13-38, 1992.

59. Glassman A. Nicotine addiction and depression. *Audio-Digest Psychiatry* 21(8), 1992.

60. Roffer-Tarlov S, Graybiel AM. Weaver mutation has differential effects on the dopamine-containing innervation of the limbic and non-limbic striatum. *Nature* 307: 62-66, 1984.

61. Bannon MJ, Reinhard JF, Bunney EB, Roth RH. Unique response to antipsychotic drugs is due to absence of terminal autoreceptors in mesocortical dopamine neurons. *Nature* 296: 444-446, 1982.

62. Glassman A. Nicotine addiction and depression. *Audio-Digest Psychiatry* 21(8), 1992.

63. Goff DC, Henderson DC, Amico E. Cigarette smoking in schizophrenia: relationship to psychopathology and medication side effects. *Am J Psychiatry* 149(9): 1189-1194, 1992.

64. White FJ, Wang RY. A10 dopamine neurons: role of autoreceptors in determining firing rate and sensitivity to dopamine agonists. *Life Sci* 34: 1161-1170, 1984.

65. Vaccarino AL, Marek P, Sternberg W, Liebeskind JC. NMDA receptor antagonist MK-801 blocks non-opioid stress-induced analgesia in the formalin test. *Pain* 50: 119-123, 1992.

66. Americ SP. Personal communication, 1992.

67. Abraham GE, Flechas JD. Management of fibromyalgia: rationale for the use of magnesium and malic acid. *J Nutr Med* 3: 49-59, 1992.

68. Pow DV. NADPH-diaphorase (nitric oxide synthase) staining in the rat supraoptic nucleus is activity-dependent: possible functional implications. *J Neuroendocrinol* 4(4): 377-379, 1992.

69. Kent S, Bluthe R-M, Kelley KW, Dantzer R. Sickness behavior as a new target for drug development. *Trends Pharmacol Sci* 13(1): 24-29, 1992.

70. Rothwell NJ. Functions and mechanisms of interleukin-1 in the brain. *Trends Pharmacol Sci* 12(11): 430-436, 1991.

71. Russell IJ, Vaeroy H, Javors M, Nyberg F. Cerebrospinal fluid biogenic amine metabolites in fibromyalgia/fibrositis syndrome and rheumatoid arthritis. *Arthritis Rheum* 35(5): 550-556, 1992.

72. Demitrack MA, Gold PW, Dale JK, Krahn DD, Kling MA, Straus SE. Plasma and cerebrospinal monoamine metabolism in patients with chronic fatigue syndrome: preliminary findings. *Biol Psychiatry* 32:1065-1077, 1992.

73. deSouza E. Personal communication, 1992.

74. Vaeroy H, Helle R, Forre O, Kass E, Terenius L. Elevated CSF levels of substance P and high incidence of Raynaud's phenomenon in patients with fibromyalgia: new features for diagnosis. *Pain* 32: 21-26, 1988.

75. Kent S, Bluthe R-M, Kelley KW, Dantzer R. Sickness behavior as a new target for drug development. *Trends Pharmacol Sci* 13(1): 24-29, 1992.

76. Lloyd A, Hickie I, Brockman A, Dwyer J, Wakefield D. Cytokine levels in serum and cerebrospinal fluid in patients with chronic fatigue syndrome and control subjects. *J Infect Dis* 164(5): 1023-1024, 1991.

77. Chelbi-Alix MK, Chousterman S. Ethanol induces 2',5'-oligoadenylate synthetase and antiviral activities through interferon-beta production. *J Biol Chem* 267(3): 1741-1745, 1992.

78. Poutsiaka DD, Clark BD, Vannier E, Dinarello CA. Production of interleukin-1 receptor antagonist and interleukin-1 beta by peripheral blood mononuclear cells is differentially regulated. *Blood* 78(5): 1275-1281, 1991.

79. da Cunha A, Vitkovic L. Transforming growth factor-beta 1 (TGF-beta 1) expression and regulation in rat cortical astrocytes. *J Neuroimmunol* 36:157-169, 1992.

80. Dinarello CA. Interleukin-1 and interleukin-1 antagonism. *Blood* 77(8): 1627-1652, 1991.

81. Chao CC, Janoff EN, Hu S, Thomas K, Gallagher M, Tsong M, Peterson PK. Altered cytokine release in peripheral blood mononuclear cell cultures from patients with the chronic fatigue syndrome. *Cytokine* 3(4): 292-298, 1991.

82. Naz RK, Kumar R. Transforming growth factor beta 1 enhances expression of 50KDz protein related to 2'-5' oligoadenylate synthetase in human sperm cells. *J Cell Physiol* 146(1): 156-163, 1991.

83. Hovanessian AG. Interferon-induced and double-stranded RNA-activated enzymes: a specific protein kinase and 2',5' oligoadenylate synthetase. *J Interferon Res* 11(4): 199-205, 1991.

84. Suhadolnik RJ, Li SW, Sobol RW, Varnum JM. 2',5' A synthetase: allosteric activation by fructose 1,6-biphosphate. *Biochem Biophys Res Comm* 169(3): 1198-1203, 1990.

85. Brady LS, Lynn AB, Whitfield HJ, Kim H, Herkenham M. Intrahippocampal colchicine alters hypothalamic corticotropin-releasing hormone and hippocampal steroid receptor mRNA in rat brain. *Neuroendocrinology* 55: 121-133, 1992.

86. Hubbell HR, Sheetz PC, Ingal SS, Brodsky I, Kariko K, Li SW, Suhadolnik RJ, Sobol RW. Heterogeneous nuclear RNA from hairy cell leukemia patients activate 2',5'-oligoadenylate synthetase: *Anticancer Res* 11(5): 1927-1932, 1991.

87. Handgretinger R, Druchelt G, Kimig A, Lang P, Daurer B, Dopfr R, Treuner J, Niephammer D. In vitro and in vivo effect of interleukin-2 on the 2',5'-oligoadenylate synthetase activity of peripheral mononuclear blood cells. *J Interferon Res* 10(I): 75-82, 1991.

88. Witt PL, Spear GT, Helgeson DO, Lindstrom MJ, Smallery RV, Borden EC. Basal and interferon induced 2',5'-oligoadenylate synthetase in human monocytes, lymphocytes, and peritoneal macrophages. *J Interferon Res* 10(4): 393-402,1990.

89. Wietzerbin J, Gaudelet C, Catinot L, Chebath J, Falcoff R. Synergistic effect of interferon-gamma and tumor necrosis factor-alpha on antiviral activity and (2'-5') oligo(A) synthetase induction in a myelomonocytic cell line. *J Leukoc Biol* 48(2): 149-155, 1990.

90. Pequegnat W, Garrick MA, Stover E. Neuroscience findings in AIDS: a review of the research sponsored by the National Institute of Mental Health. *Prog Neuro-Psychopharmacol Biol Psychiatry* 16: 145-170, 1992.

91. Caplan JD, Sharma T, Rosenblum LA, Friedman S, Bassoff TB, Barbour RL, Gorman JM. Effects of sodium lactate infusion on cisternal lactate and carbon dioxide levels in nonhuman primates. *Am J Psychiatry* 149(10): 1369-1373, 1992.

92. Goldman-Rakic PS. Prefrontal cortical dysfunction in schizophrenia: the relevance of working memory. In: Carroll BJ, Barnett JE (eds.). *Psychopathology and the Brain.* New York, Raven Press, 1991.

93. Insel TR. Toward a neuroanatomy of obsessive-compulsive disorder. *Arch Gen Psychiatry* 49: 739-744, 1992.

94. Modele JG, Mountz JM, Curtis G, Greden J. Neurophysiologic dysfunction in basal ganglia/limbic striatal and thalamo-cortical circuits as a pathogenetic mechanism of obsessive-compulsive disorder. *J Neuropsychiatry* 1: 27-36, 1989.

95. Ichise M, Salit IE, Abbey SE, Chung D-C, Gray B, Kirsch JC, Freedman M. Assessment of regional cerebral perfusion in ^{99m}Tc-HMPAO SPECT in chronic fatigue syndrome. *Nuc Med Comm* 13: 767-772, 1992.

96. Mountz JM, Mountz JD, Modele JG. Decreased caudate activity measured by ^{99m}Tc-HMPAO brain SPECT in fibromyalgia. *Arth Rheum* 35 (9): S113, 1992.

97. Broder GE, Stewart JW, Towey JP, Friedman D, Tenke CE, Voglmaier MM, Leite P, Cohen P, Quitkin FM. Abnormal cerebral laterality in bipolar depression: convergence of behavioral and brain event-related potential findings. *Biol Psychiatry* 32: 33-47, 1992.

98. Weinberger DR, Berman KF, Suddath R, Fuller-Torrey E. Evidence of dysfunction of a prefrontal-limbic network in schizophrenia: a magnetic resonance imaging and regional cerebral blood flow study of discordant monozygotic twins. *Am J Psychiatry* 149(7): 890-897, 1992.

Addendum I:
Transneuronal Retrograde Messengers in Chronic Fatigue Syndrome

Low dose sublingual nitroglycerin (NTG) works best on the symptoms of CFS patients with fibromyalgia (FM) and has a greater effect on women than men. The most pronounced result is relief of fibromyalgic pain and tenderness and sometimes headaches, which do not seem to be related to FM. NTG also reliably relieves the "idiopathic" chest pain which CFS patients experience. Some patients report that NTG potentiates the effect and duration of opioid analgesics significantly although there is nothing in the literature as of this writing on the interaction of NO and opioids. NTG is often remarkably effective in relieving the pain of deafferentation syndrome and reflex sympathetic dystrophy, two rather intractable disorders that may have a basis in limbic dysfunction.[1] NTG will sometimes relieve the pain of irritable bowel syndrome;[2] this relief is usually accompanied by anxiolysis. Sore throats are sometimes ameliorated by NO, also. Little has been written about the effect of NO on pain. That which has, suggests an association with intrathecal NMDA-mediated *hyper*algesia[3.] NO inhibitors and NMDA antagonists are being developed as analgesics. NO apparently has a different effect in FM supraspinal networks than it does at the spinal cord level.

An alteration in mood is commonly reported. Usually the patient feels more relaxed. Sometimes the patient is sedated. Depression is

[DocuSerial™ co-indexing entry]

"Addendum I: Transneuronal Retrograde Messengers in Chronic Fatigue Syndrome," Goldstein, J.A. Published in: *Haworth Library of the Medical Neurobiology of Somatic Disorders* (The Haworth Medical Press), Volume 1, 1993 and *Chronic Fatigue Syndromes: The Limbic Hypothesis*, Goldstein, J.A., The Haworth Medical Press, 1993.

often relieved. Many patients feel mildly intoxicated. A number feel overstimulated, or "antsy," and transient euphoria is occasionally experienced. Dysphoria or intense overstimulation occurs rarely.

How might the reported improvement in symptoms after NTG administration be explained from information provided about the pluripotential effects of this transneuronal retrograde messenger? NO may have an anxiolytic effect. A NO synthesis inhibitor can block behaviors induced by chlordiazepoxide in mice. This effect can be reversed by L-arginine.[4] NO synthase is colocalized with GABA in the substantia gelatinosa of rat spinal cord.[5] Patients report that the quality of NTG-induced anxiolysis is different from that obtained from benzodiazepines. They report feeling less drugged, and thus more "normal." Relief of depression and/or production of behavioral stimulation may be related to the facilitatory role that NO plays in dopamine release,[6] which is not NMDA-mediated. NMDA does enhance NO synthase by increasing the influx of calcium and its binding to calmodulin. Calcium ionophores such as 3,4-diaminopyridine might thus be effective treatments for CFS. Hanbauer et al. suggest that NO . . . "might serve as a diffusible signal within neuronal tissue that is necessary for the release of catecholamines and possibly other neurotransmitters evoked from axonal terminals. This proposed function for NO would be an addition to the three roles for the substance in vertebrate nervous systems, . . . that is, regulation of local blood flow, regulation of synaptic efficacy, and segregation of axonal arbors on the basis of neural activity."[7]

An increase in energy, relief of fatigue, and a sensation of "I feel much lighter" are often described after the first dose of NTG in CFS patients. It is difficult to assign a neurotransmitter role to these improvements. Currently, I would ascribe them to an improvement in limbic integrative function on a neuronal network basis. If neuronal excitability is involved in this process, NO might be inhibitory in the hippocampal, striatal, cerebellar and amygdala neurons.[8] Vision is often brighter and less blurred after NTG. cGMP synthesis in on-bipolar cells is catalyzed by NO-sensitive cyclase,[9] and visual brightening and enhancement of color perception could occur through this mechanism.

Many patients complain of air hunger or dyspnea, with normal pulmonary function tests. This symptom is almost always relieved by NTG. This result may be related to amygdala neurons in the cortical nuclei that are NADPH-diaphorase positive. These same neurons are thought to be cholinergic, and resemble neurons that contain somatostatin and neuropeptide Y.[10] CFS patients who respond to NTG often report a clearing of "brain fog" and an increased ability to read and remember. NO is well known to be involved in long-term potentiation, and has been shown to play a role in spatial learning in rats and conditioned eyeblink response in rabbits.[11]

CFS patients with multiple chemical sensitivity (MCS) sometimes report improvement in their symptoms after NTG. In one experiment, odorant-induced cGMP response was thought to be NO-mediated in the Sprague-Dawley rat.[12] Some MCS patients are not improved by NTG. It is possible that they may have a deficiency of another transneuronal retrograde messenger, carbon monoxide (CO). The olfactory tubercle in rats in another study was found to lack NO synthase, but to be enriched in heme oxygenase-2, which produces CO from heme, and guanylyl cyclase, which is stimulated by CO as well as NO.[13] Heme oxygenase-2 is present in high concentrations in the brain, although the reason for its being there was enigmatic until recently.[14,15] CO is a vasodilator, although much less potent than NO.[16] I am tempted to think that the regional cerebral hypoperfusion of some of our CFS patients may be due to a decreased regional stimulation of heme oxygenase-2. We have seen normalization of hypoperfused areas on brain SPECT in CFS patients who respond to NO, with no effect on rCBF elsewhere, suggesting a localized NO deficit in these responders.[17]

How to increase brain CO is problematic. Heme oxygenase-2, in contrast to heme oxygenase-1, is not inducible.[18] It would be possibly hazardous to have patients inhale low concentrations of CO, which avidly binds to hemoglobin, although not as avidly as NO.[19] A CFS patient who fell ill in Lake Tahoe in 1985 reported a six-month remission after inhaling exhaust fumes from his racing car. Could this improvement have been due to CO? Certainly not all patients would respond to CO, since I have evaluated ill CFS patients who smoked cigarettes and had elevated carboxyhemoglobins.

Low central levels of NO in CFS should reflect decreased concentrations of EAAs. CFS quinolinic acid and a related metabolite, kynurenic acid, were measured in a variety of neurologic disorders, including CFS.[20] Quinolinic acid is an endogenous NMDA agonist synthesized from L-tryptophan, and kynurenic acid is an NMDA antagonist. Very small increases in quinolinic acid and neopterin were found in patients with CFS (n=18), suggesting immune activation. Glutamate was not measured. Patients with depression were normal in all measured variables. I am not sure yet how this finding relates to my postulated CFS glutamate deficiency. It is certainly possible that subgroups of CFS (especially those who feel worse after NTG) could have elevated concentrations of NO, glutamate, and possibly IL-1 beta and other cytokines. The quinolinic acid results in CFS should be confirmed by using larger samples and measuring more EAAs. Elevated quinolinic acid may be related to the tendency of central alpha interferon to shunt tryptophan into the kynurenine pathway.

The most vexing problem in my use of NTG in CFS has been the development of tolerance, which is sometimes extremely rapid, occurring even after the first dose. Often the development of neurological tolerance seems dissociated from cardiovascular tolerance, since adverse reactions secondary to vasodilatation usually continue. Furthermore, many NTG-tolerant CFS patients never regain any NTG efficacy no matter how long they refrain from its use. I have tried all suggested methods used to ameliorate NTG tolerance in cardiac patients, including the –SH donors methionine and n-acetyl cysteine, but they are not usually effective. It is thought that sulfhydryl groups are involved in the enzymatic conversion of NTG to NO. There are experimental drugs which produce NO to which tolerance does not develop in cardiac patients, but I have not yet tried them in CFS. I have not yet tried precursor and cofactor loading with L-arginine, malic acid (to increase NADPH), tetrahydrobiopterin (which is not well absorbed orally), and flavin nucleotides. This approach seems feasible to me, however.

Although increasing brain NO in CFS is novel and exciting, it is somewhat like using beta-agonists to treat asthma—it does not get at the root of the problem. Perhaps we can trace NO pathways to better understand CFS pathophysiologic mechanisms.

REFERENCES

1. Melzack R. Phantom limbs. *Sci Am* 266(4):120-127, 1992.

2. Saffrey MJ, Hassall CJS, Hoyle CHV, et al. Colocalization of nitric oxide synthase and NADPH-diaphorase in cultured myenteric neurones. *NeuroReport* 3:333-336, 1992.

3. Kitto KF, Haley JE, Wilcox GL. Involvement of nitric oxide in spinally mediated hyperalgesia in the mouse. *Neurosci Lett* 148:1-5, 1992.

4. Quock RM, Nguyen E. Possible involvement of nitric oxide in chlordiazepoxide-induced anxiolysis in mice. *Life Sciences* 51:PL 255-260, 1992.

5. Valtschanoff JG, Weinberg RJ, Rustioni A, Schmidt HHHW. Nitric oxide synthase and GABA colocalize in lamina II of rat spinal cord. *Neurosci Lett* 148:6-10, 1992.

6. Hanbauer I, Wink D, Osawa Y, Edelman G, Gally GA. Role of nitric oxide in NMDA-evoked release of [^{3}H]-dopamine from striatal slices. *NeuroReport* 3:409-412, 1992.

7. Hanbauer I, Wink D, Osawa Y, Edelman G, Gally GA. Role of nitric oxide in NMDA-evoked release of [^{3}H]-dopamine from striatal slices. *NeuroReport* 3:409-412, 1992.

8. Rondouin G, Lerner-Natoli M, Manzoni O, Lafon-Cazal M. Bockaert J. A nitric oxide (NO) synthase inhibitor accelerates amygdala kindling. *NeuroReport* 3:805-808, 1992.

9. Shiells R, Falk G. Retinal on-bipolar cells contain a nitric-oxide sensitive guanylate cyclase. *NeuroReport* 3:845-848, 1992.

10. McDonald AJ, Payne DR, Mascagni F. Identification of putative nitric oxide producing neurons in the rat amygdala using NADPH-diaphorase histochemistry. *Neuroscience* 52(1):97-106, 1993.

11. Chapman PF, Atkins CM, Allen MT, Haley JE, Steinmetz JE. Inhibition of nitric oxide synthesis impairs two different forms of learning. *NeuroReport* 3:567-570, 1992.

12. Breer B, Klemm T, Boekhoff I. Nitric oxide mediated formation of cyclic GMP in the olfactory system. *NeuroReport* 3:1030-1033, 1992.

13. Verma A, Hirsch DJ, Glatt CE, Ronnett GV, Snyder SH. Carbon monoxide: a putative neural messenger. *Science* 259:381-384, 1993.

14. Sun Y, Rotenberg M, Maines MD. Developmental expression of heme oxygenase isoenzymes in rat brain: two HO-2 mRNAs are detected. *J Biol Chem* 265 (14):8212-8217, 1990.

15. Marks GS, Brien JF, Nakatsu K, McLaughlin BE. Does carbon monoxide have a physiological function? *Trends Pharmacol Sci* 12:185-188, 1991.

16. Furchgott RF, Jothiandan D. Endothelium-dependent and -independent vasodilatation involving cyclic GMP: relaxation induced by nitric oxide, carbon monoxide and light. *Blood Vessels* 28:52-61, 1991.

17. Schachter BA. Heme catabolism by heme oxygenase: physiology, regulation, and mechanism of function. *Sem Hematol* 25(4): 349-369, 1988.

18. Marks GS, Brien JF, Nakatsu K, McLaughlin BE. Does carbon monoxide have a physiological function? *Trends Pharmacol Sci* 12:185-188, 1991.

19. Goadsby PJ, Kaube H, Hoskink L. Nitric oxide synthesis couples cerebral blood flow and metabolism. *Brain Res* 595:167-170, 1992.

20. Heyes MP, Saito K, Crowley JS, et al. Quinolinic acid and kynurenine pathway metabolism in inflammatory and non-inflammatory neurological disease. *Brain* 115:1249-1273, 1992.

APPENDIX

Neuropharmacology of Chronic Fatigue Syndrome

1. H-2 blockers:
   ranitidine (Zantac): 150 mg BID
   cimetidine (Tagamet): 400 mg BID.
   a. modulate cytokines via suppressor T cells
   b. modulate histaminergic neurotransmission

2. Cyclic antidepressants, daily doses:
   doxepin (Sinequan) capsules and elixir: 2-300 mg HS
   amitriptyline (Elavil): 10-300 mg HS-therapeutic blood
      levels valid
   cyclobenzaprine (Flexeril): 5-10 mg HS to 10 mg TID
   imipramine (Tofranil): 10-300 mg HS-therapeutic blood
      levels valid
   nortriptyline (Pamelor): 10-150 mg HS-therapeutic window
   desipramine (Norpramin): 10-300 mg HS-therapeutic blood
      levels valid

[DocuSerial™ co-indexing entry]

"Appendix," Goldstein, J.A. Published in: *Haworth Library of the Medical Neurobiology of Somatic Disorders* (The Haworth Medical Press), Volume 1, 1993 and *Chronic Fatigue Syndromes: The Limbic Hypothesis,* Goldstein, J.A., The Haworth Medical Press, 1993.

protriptylene (Vivactil): 5-10 mg HS-for sleep apnea; 10-60 mg as antidepressant

amoxapine (Asendin): 50-400 mg HS-observe for tardive dyskinesia;

clomipramine (Anafranil): 25-200 mg QD

3. Selective serotonin reuptake inhibitors (SSRI):
    a. fluoxetine (Prozac): 1-80 mg QD.
        Possible therapeutic window in depression. Comes in elixir for easy dosage titration.
    b. sertraline (Zoloft): 50-200 mg QD.
        2-week period of metabolic elimination more rapid than fluoxetine (5-6 weeks). May have superior adverse reaction profile.
    c. paroxetine (Paxil): 20-50 mg QD.

4. Bupropion (Wellbutrin): 200-450 mg QD.
    In doses at least 4-6 hours apart. Do not give more than 150 mg in a single dose. Risk of seizure overrated. No similar antidepressant. Mild dopamine agonist.
    Diethylpropion (Tenuate):
    May work in a similar manner.

5. Buspirone (Buspar):
    A 5HT-1A agonist, which is a property shared by SSRIs. Buspirone raises prolactin in CFS compared to major depression possibly indicating hypersensitivity of the 5HT-1A receptor. Not effective for panic disorder. Dose: 10-60 mg QD.

6. Lithium carbonate:
    A serotoninergic anti-kindling agent of little use in CFS.

7. Monamine oxidase inhibitors (MAOI):
    The most effective pharmacotherapy for atypical depression. "The atom bomb for panic disorder."
    a. Non-selective:
        1. Phenelzine (Nardil): 45-90 mg QD
           reduce dose after response is obtained. Avoid tyramine, found in wine, cheese, and aged food. Avoid certain medications: SSRIs, sumatriptan, adrenergic agents,

buspirone, bupropion, opioids, especially meperidine (Demerol) and dextromethorphan. Sublingual nifedipine 10 mg prn hypertensive headache.

2. Isocarboxazid (Marplan): 10-30 mg per day–10-20 mg per day once response is obtained.

3. Tranylcypromine (Parnate): 10-60 mg per day.
   Less sedating, less weight gain, possible withdrawal symptoms if dose greater than 60 mg per day.

b. Selective
   1. Selegiline (Eldepryl):
      MAO Type B inhibitor. Loses specificity if given in doses > 10 mg per day.

8. Antidepressant potentiation:
   a. CA + SSRI
   b. CA + LiCO$_3$
   c. CA + buspirone
   d. CA + thyroid
   e. CA + MAOI + (?) stimulant
   f. LiCO$_3$ + MAOI
   g. Thyroid + MAOI
   h. LiCO$_3$ + bupropion
   i. CA + bupropion
   j. Thyroid + bupropion
   k. SSRI + thyroid
   l. SSRI + LiCO$_3$
   m. SSRI + buspirone

9. Benzodiazepines (BDZ):
   a. Alprazolam (Xanax): 5-6 mg per day is usual dose for treatment of panic disorder. An effective antidepressant.
   b. Clonazepam (Klonopin): An antikindling agent as well as an anti-anxiety agent.
   c. Lorazepam (Ativan) IM or IV to diagnose panic attack.
      Physician must make risk/benefit determination regarding chronic use of BDZ. Often combined with antidepressants and also used as hypnotics.

10. Trazodone (Desyrel): 50-600 mg HS.
    Probably more effective as a hypnotic than as an antidepressant. May be added to MAOIs.

11. Antikindling agents:
    a. Carbamazepine (Tegretol)
       Of little value in CFS.
    b. Valproate (Depakote):
       Effective in panic disorder, migraine, and post-traumatic stress disorder.
    c. Phenytoin (Dilantin):
       Of little value in CFS.

12. Nitroglycerin and derivatives, converted to nitric oxide. Dose: 0.04-0.15 mg sublingual nitroglycerin.
    Most benefit in patients with fibromyalgia. Possibly useful as a pharmacologic probe. L-arginine and tetrahydrobiopterin, as well as agents which enhance NADPH production, may increase the biosynthesis of nitric oxide or increase the activity of nitric oxide synthase, shown to be NADPH-diaphorase.

13. Neuroleptics and atypical neuroleptics such as clozapine (Clozaril), and rispiridone are of little value in CFS. CFS patients may be unusually apt to develop extrapyramidal symptoms.

14. Calcium channel blockers, especially nimodipine (Nimotop), 30-60 mg TID.
    Dihydropyridines have the best effect. Certain patients may have improved cognition and increased energy with nimodipine. Tolerance may develop to nimodipine.

15. Adamantan compounds:
    a. Amantadine:
       useful in multiple sclerosis for pain and fatigue in dose of 200-300 mg per day. Possibly effective in SSRI-induced anorgasmia. May help flu-like symptoms and sore throats in CFS. A dopamine agonist.

b. Kemantan:

claimed to be successful in treating CFS by Dr. N. Artzimovich in Moscow. Not available at present.

16. Other serotonin agents:

a. Ondansetron (Zofran):

a $5HT_3$ receptor antagonist used as an antiemetic. An oral form is undergoing clinical trials in various psychiatric disorders. It has not helped other symptoms in my nauseated CFS patients.

b. Fenfluramine (Pondimin):

an anorectic agent which is a generalized serotonin agonist. Raises CRH levels. Not effective in CFS, even when combined with the vasopressin derivative DDAVP, which also increases CRH levels.

c. Ritanserin:

a $5HT_{1c}/5HT_2$ antagonist. Appeared effective in an open fibromyalgia study. Some patients in this population had withdrawal symptoms, never before reported with this agent. Experimental.

17. Stimulants:

a. methylphenidate (Ritalin)
b. dextroamphetamine (Dexedrine)
c. pemoline (Cylert):

Although used in the HIV cognitive/motor complex, they are only mildly effective in CFS.

18. Thymopentin (TP5):

A thymic peptide, experimental in the USA, which is a CRH agonist.

19. S-adenosylmethionine (SAMe): 600-1600 mg per day as an oral medication.

A methyl group donor used as an antiarthritic, analgesic, and antidepressant in Europe for almost ten years. Found effective in two double-blind, placebo-controlled studies in fibromyalgia. Not available in the USA. Vitamin B_{12} may act in CFS via SAMe.

20. Essential fatty acids:
    Enhance the production of prostaglandins which are intermediates in the stimulation of CRH secretion by IL-6.

21. Pyridostigmine (Mestinon):
    May increase strength and decrease fatigue in CFS patients with myasthenic presentation. Increases the secretion of growth hormone, low in CFS/FM.

22. Ampligen, lentinan, kutapressin:
    May increase central IL-1 levels.

23. Light therapy: for winter depression and for sleep phase disorder.
    a. Sleeping too late: bright light exposure when waking is desired.
    b. Waking too early: bright light in the late afternoon or evening.

24. Acetazolamide (Diamox):
    Sometimes effective for pressure headaches. Causes paresthesias. Occasionally other CFS symptoms respond as well.

25. Cognition-enhancing agents:
    Many not available in USA. Most do not work very well in CFS.
    a. ergoloid mesylates (Hydergine) 9-12 mg per day.
    b. tacrine-cholinergic agonist: it and similar agents may be effective in CFS by increasing limbic acetylcholine levels and stimulating the production of nitric oxide.
    c. nootropics: piracetam, oxiracetam, aniracetam
    d. acetylcarnitine: perhaps works as an acetyl-group donor
    e. nerve growth factor (NGF)-may be low in CFS.
    f. lecithin (phosphatidylcholine)
    g. gangliosides

   h.   vinpocetine
   i.   glycosaminoglycans

26. Maxillary splint to alter trigeminal nerve input into the limbic
     system–an experimental device.

27. Very low-dose opioids:
     Some patients feel well for 1-2 days by taking one Darvocet-
     N. This treatment may work by a multi-synaptic pathway
     involving hypersensitive mu-opioid receptors, which may
     stimulate the secretion of catecholamines and serotonin.

28. Capsaicin (Zostrix):
     An agent which inhibits substance P neurotransmission when
     used topically. Mildly effective for pain in CFS/FM. Used in
     post-herpetic neuralgia, peripheral neuropathies, and arthri-
     tis.

29. Intravenous immunoglobulin:
     Some patients became euphoric or hypomanic after adminis-
     tration. Used in treatment-resistant epilepsy of childhood.

30. Peptide T:
     An agent which has had successful therapeutic trials in AIDS.
     Blocks the VIP/CD4 receptor. May work as a VIP agonist to
     increase central IL-1 levels. Some CFS patients have been
     helped by this agent. We hope to do a controlled experiment
     in CFS using Peptide T.

31. Cognitive-behavioral therapy:
     Improves abnormal elevations in caudate nucleus metabolic
     activity seen in PET scans of patients with obsessive-compul-
     sive disorder. May alter neurotransmission in other syn-
     dromes, could increase the number of pre-synaptic vesicles
     in certain networks, and could otherwise change neuronal
     biology and cortical architecture.

32. DHEA (dehydroepiandrosterone):
    An adrenal steroid possibly of benefit in CFS. Some CFS patients have low levels of DHEA sulfate. Secretion regulated by unknown hypothalamic factor, apparently not CRH or ACTH. Not FDA approved. Produced in brain glial cells and regulated independently of peripheral secretion.

33. Pregnenolone:
    The first compound after cholesterol in steroid biosynthesis. Apparently non-toxic. It (or its congeners) may be useful in several conditions, including CFS and PMS, by further opening the chloride channel of the $GABA_A$ receptor. Experimental. DHEA and pregnenolone are two of a class of endogenously produced compounds called "neurosteroids" which should have value in CFS.

34. Coenzyme Q10:
    60-200 mg per day if mitochondrial cytochrome oxidase activity is thought to be reduced. May be combined with oral iron and vitamin B_6. This treatment has been used in Alzheimer's disease in patients with normal iron levels.

35. Transdermal nicotine patch:
    Stimulates the nicotinic cholinergic receptor and may thereby increase the activity of nitric oxide synthase. Dose is one-half of a 5 mg Nicotrol (Parke-Davis) patch daily.

36. Somatostatin octreotide (Sandostatin):
    0.05 mg will sometimes relieve headaches and pain within 30 minutes. It may then be given in a QD or BID subcutaneous dose. Sometimes other symptoms will respond, as well.

37. Sympathomimetic ophthalmic solutions:
    a. naphazoline HCl 0.1%
    b. epinephrine 1:1000
    c. dipivefrin HCl 0.1%
    d. apraclonidine.

e. phenylephrine

These agents work rapidly and naphazoline is the first treatment I try on most new patients. Their spectrum of action is similar to nitroglycerin. They also may help nasal congestion, asthma, and ventricular premature beats.

38. Proparacaine HCl 0.5%:

A useful agent for central pain conditions such as trigeminal neuralgia, atypical facial pain, some cases of fibromyalgia, and other types of central pain. Duration of action is from one hour to two weeks. It may damage the cornea if used more than twice weekly.

39. Insulin-like growth factor 1 (Somatomedin-C):

May be a useful treatment for CFS/FM.

Chronic Fatigue Syndrome Institute

Jay A. Goldstein, M.D.

SCREENING PSYCHOLOGICAL REPORT

Name: _____ Date: _____ Age: _____ Sex: _____

The following instruments were administered:

Symptom Checklist 90:

The Symptom Checklist 90 is a 90-item, 5-point self-rating scale. It has 9 dimensional scales: somatization, obsessive-compulsive, interpersonal sensitivity, depression, anxiety, hostility, phobic anxiety, paranoid ideation, and psychoticism.

Global Severity Index: _____

Positive Symptom Distress Index: _____

Positive Symptom Total: _____

Refer to the enclosed report.

Interpretation: _____

_____

_____

Beck Depression Inventory:

The Beck Depression Inventory is a 63-item, 4-point self-rating scale indicative of a person's feelings during the past week including today.

0-9 normal/asymptomatic
10-18 mild - moderate depression
19-29 moderate - severe depression
30-63 extremely severe depression

This person's score was _____ indicating_____

Items marked as 3 on a scale of 0 to 3 include:_____

_____

Interpretation:_____

         _____

         _____

Beck Anxiety Inventory

The Beck Anxiety Inventory is a 21-item, 4-point adjective self-rating scale that indicates the severity of anxiety felt during the past week, including today. It gives an estimate of the overall severity of the person's anxiety, with a maximum score of 63.

0-9   normal
10-18 mild - moderate anxiety
19-29 moderate - severe anxiety
30-63 severe anxiety

Total scores for women with anxiety disorder may be an average of 4 points higher than those for men with anxiety disorder. Younger patients report more anxiety than older patients. The items can be clustered into 4 subscales: Neurophysiological, subjective, panic, and autonomic.

This person's score was _____, indicating _____

Items marked as 3 on a scale of 0 to 3 include: _____

_____

Most items of significance fell in the subscale category: ─────────

Interpretation: _____

_____

_____

Analysis of the **Karnofsky Performance Scale** (0 to 100) indicates this person rates self at _____:

Interpretation: _____

_____

_____

Analysis of the **Somatosensory Amplification Scale** indicates this person views self as:

_____

_____

_____

_____ Meets _____ does not meet **Columbia Criteria** for probable or definite atypical depression:

a. Mood reactivity when depressed:
b. Has two (one for probable) associated features: hyperphagia, hypersomnia, leaden paralysis and pathologic sensitivity to interpersonal rejection as a trait through adulthood.

Further Comment: _____

_____

_____

Summary:

_____

_____

_____

_____

Recommendations:

    (1) Further neuropsychological testing including structured interview.
    (2) Functional capacity evaluation.
    (3) Disability evaluation.
    (4) Psychotherapy.
    (5) Other:_____

Addendum II:
Is Chronic Fatigue Syndrome a Disorder of the Central Neurogenic Regulation of Cerebral Circulation?

It is possible that chronic fatigue syndrome (CFS) symptoms are a manifestation of regional cerebral ischemia produced by a dysregulated neural network. Current dogma holds that cerebral metabolic activity is coupled to regional blood flow (rCBF). A key coupling compound to effect this linkage is nitric oxide (NO).[1,2] Thus, when neuronal firing increases, so does rCBF, by neuronal and/or glial regulation of local nitric oxide synthase. The endothelial cell may also be involved "as a transducer of neurogenic influences in the vascular system."[3]

Such a system may not always be involved in the rCBF changes seen in CFS and related disorders. Rather than rCBF being primarily determined by local metabolic needs, it may be regulated (or dysregulated) by a central neurogenic mechanism. Autonomic ganglia in the head and neck such as the sphenopalatine, superior cervical, ciliary, otic and the internal carotid plexus, all influence rCBF. NO may act as a transmitter between pre- and post-ganglionic sympathetic neurons.[4] NO is found in neurons of the rostral ventral medulla, and may aid in integration of somatosensory input with autonomic regulation.[5] Cranial nerves such as the trigeminal, facial, glossopharyngeal, and vagus also regulate rCBF. The locus cer-

[DocuSerial™ co-indexing entry]

"Addendum II: Is Chronic Fatigue Syndrome a Disorder of the Central Neurogenic Regulation of Cerebral Circulation?," Goldstein, J.A. Published in: *Haworth Library of the Medical Neurobiology of Somatic Disorders* (The Haworth Medical Press), Volume 1, 1993 and *Chronic Fatigue Syndromes: The Limbic Hypothesis,* Goldstein, J.A., The Haworth Medical Press, 1993.

uleus, raphe nuclei, nucleus basalis/fastigial nucleus regulate norepinephrine, serotonin, and acetylcholine secretion respectively.[6] Other vasoactive transmitters include neuropeptide Y (NPY), endothelin, protein kinase C, vasoactive intestinal peptide (VIP) and related peptides, angiotensin II, substance P (SP)/neurokinin A, interleukin-1 beta, prostacyclin, thromboxane, other vasodilator prostaglandins, bradykinin, interleukin-1 receptor antagonist (IRA), histamine, ATP, adenosine, and calcitonin gene-related peptide (CGRP). The sphenopalatine ganglia have the highest concentration of nitric oxide synthase (NOS) and VIP immunoreactivity. Recall that VIP may induce IL-1 beta. In the trigeminal ganglion, nitric oxide synthase-immunoreactivity (NOS-IR) is found primarily in the ophthalmic division, but is not colocalized with CGRP. Nerve fibers may serve as a non-endothelial source of NO.

NPY is also found in the sphenopalatine ganglia in large concentrations, as is choline acetyltransferase. NOS-IR axons which innervate the rostral circle of Willis project mainly from the sphenopalatine ganglion.[7] The trigeminal nerve sends branches to the sphenopalatine and ciliary ganglia. Norepinephrine, NPY, endothelin, thromboxane, IRA, angiotensin II and protein kinase C are vasoconstrictors in cerebral vessels.[8,9,10] The other transmitters are vasodilators, except for serotonin, which can be either, depending upon its local concentration and the receptors involved.

We have noted in brain SPECT of CFS patients that decreased rCBF is induced by a variety of stressful stimuli, including exercise, calculations, and spraying perfume in the room. The decrease is usually quite marked, occurs rapidly, and correlates with worsening of symptoms. When we compare SPECT and PET in the same patients, the SPECT abnormalities are usually much more profound and do not necessarily correspond to the hypometabolism noted on PET. SPECT measures only rCBF, while PET measures the metabolism of fluorideoxyglucose in the brain, which is assumed to reflect rCBF.

At least half of my patients have a major improvement in symptoms within 5 to 30 minutes after taking nitroglycerin, nimodipine, or sympathomimetic ophthalmic drops such as naphazoline 0.1% (Albalon, Vasocon, etc.), apraclonidine (Iopidine), phenylephrine 2.5%, dipivefrine (Propine) or epinephrine 1:1000. Muscarinic agonists occasionally work like sympathomimetics; antagonists are not usually effective, although pilocarpine will occasionally be of benefit. Prostaglandin antagonists ameliorate ciliary spasm (from photophobia) only, and proparacaine 0.5% is effective primarily for central pain disorders.

I reasoned that sympathomimetic ophthalmic drops probably worked by stimulating the trigeminal-cerebrovascular system to secrete SP or CGRP which counteract pathogenic vasoconstriction.[11,12] If the drops are effective, a CFS patient has similar beneficial responses as obtained from nitroglycerin, with none of the adverse effects. Patients report feeling more alert, having more mental clarity, increased energy, less anxiety, clearer vision, and sometimes less pain. Naphazoline has relieved nasal congestion and asthmatic bronchoconstriction. I use naphazoline 0.1% first, but may try other sympathomimetics if there is lack of response, or if the duration of action of naphazoline is too short. I have been pleasantly surprised by the response of patients with treatment-resistant depression and Tourette's disorder to apraclonidine, a topical alpha-2 agonist. Instillation of ophthalmic medications has a tremendous unexplored potential for treating neuroregulatory disorders. Serotoninergic and dopaminergic ophthalmic agents are under investigation for glaucoma treatment but are not clinically available. Hydroxyamphetamine (Paredrine) is not currently marketed. Ophthalmic beta-blockers are of no benefit, and thymoxamine, an alpha adrenergic antagonist used in other countries to treat glaucoma and reverse mydriasis is not available in the United States.[13] The way these drugs, most of which are approved for the treatment of glaucoma, reduce intraocular pressure is poorly understood. Epinephrine and timolol (Timoptic) actually have opposing effects on the beta receptor. I thought there were several possible modes of action of ophthalmic neuropharmacologic agents in CFS:

1. By stimulating the trigeminal-cerebrovascular system via ophthalmic nerve fibers to the circle of Willis which secrete SP and neurokinins producing vasodilatation in regionally ischemic areas. When we perform pre- and post-treatment brain SPECT with nitroglycerin or nimodipine, we note that the hypoperfused areas tend to normalize, while areas of normal perfusion remain

about the same. Occasionally hypoperfused areas further decrease their rCBF, even though symptoms lessen.

2. Through a multisynaptic neurogenic trigeminal pathway through the pons and into the reticular formation, locus ceruleus, dorsal raphe, non-specific thalamic nuclei and then to the limbic system. If the activity of this network, particularly the reticular formation, were dysregulated, abnormalities in sensory gating could occur which could contribute to CFS pathophysiology. Trigeminal fibers could also synapse with the facial and vagus nerves through the trigeminal mesencephalic and spinal tracts. The trigeminal nerve sends branches to the sphenopalatine, ciliary and superior cervical ganglia and could thus modulate the function of these structures also.

3. By having ophthalmic drops be absorbed parenterally and thus act as intravenous agents.

4. By a combination of these, or via an as yet undiscovered pathway, perhaps involving the release of NO, or another gaseous neurotransmitter which may have a beneficial effect independent of its vasoregulatory role.

Neurobehavioral disorders may be caused by dysregulation of regional cerebral blood flow on a neurogenic basis, which, unlike a migraine aura, could persist for many years, unless the blood flow changes were epiphenomena. The ganglionic and brain stem structures involved are modulated by the posterior and lateral hypothalamus, which, of course, is modulated by the limbic system. Just as autonomic effects on peripheral tissues can be precisely regulated by unknown mechanisms in the central nervous system, so could the central autonomic circulatory effectors be specifically controlled.

Such a pathophysiology could explain sudden changes for the better or worse in patients in the normal course of their illness, and how someone who has been sick for 20 years can feel better in 30 minutes ("You mean I've been sick for all this time and all they had to do was to give me a pill?"). It could also explain why the symptoms of CFS are not only similar to temporolimbic epilepsy, but also to migraine auras. It would not explain, however, why CFS patients do not respond to potent vasodilator agents such as acetazolamide and hydralazine, or to antimigraine drugs such as propanolol.

When I see a new patient with CFS, I usually try, in order, napha-zoline, very low dose nitroglycerin, and nimodipine. None, one, two or all three of the agents may be effective. Nimodipine sometimes will not work for 5 to 7 days. Other calcium channel blockers do not work as well as nimodipine, perhaps because nimodipine binds better to ischemic areas.[14] Some of my patients have been taking nimodipine for more than four years.[15] When they try to stop, they relapse. I think nimodipine has a mode of action in CFS which distinguishes it from other calcium channel blockers. Nitrendipine, for example, raises DHEA-S levels.[16] The effects of nimodipine cannot be produced solely by arterial dilatation, since nicardipine (Cardene) is better in this regard,[17] but nicardipine is quite inferior in ameliorating CFS symptoms. Perhaps nimodipine releases NO.[18] Perhaps the NO release occurs only in certain neural networks or neuronal/glial structures.

Very little is known about the central neurogenic regulation of cerebral circulation. The idea that there could be a persistent neuro-genic regional hypoperfusion with neurobehavioral consequences appears to be a new one, but offers opportunities for further study and novel therapeutic interventions. Whether a medication causes vasodilatation or vasoconstriction in the CFS patient may be inci-dental to its therapeutic effect, and its vasoregulatory result could be due to a summation of constrictive and dilatory factors which might be, at least in part, epiphenomena.[19] Medications useful in CFS should be considered for their possible effects on the autonomic ganglia of the head and neck, since those drugs which cannot pene-trate the blood-brain barrier can still (e.g., pyridostigmine) affect these structures, and hence rCBF.

We are investigating the mode of action of naphazoline 0.1% ophthalmic solution by sequential brain SPECT. If improvement is correlated to increased rCBF by stimulation of the ophthalmic branch of the trigeminal nerve, instillation of the medication into one eye should result in ipsilateral arterial dilatation, since the tri-geminal vascular system has only an ipsilateral distribution.

Preliminary results indicate, however, that primarily ipsilateral arterial *constriction* occurs (although the patient feels better), a find-ing we did not anticipate. The mechanism for this result is obscure. The trigeminal nerve is not known to communicate with the superior cervical ganglion, the major mediator of cerebral vasoconstriction, except in the regulation of ipsilateral sweating. It could regulate the activity of the locus ceruleus and/or raphe nuclei in the brain stem, both of which could regulate rCBF. Some patients remark that naphazoline mimics the action of nitroglycerin, but four have reported that there is no additive effect, i.e., either naphazoline or nitroglycerin is effective, and combining the two treatments is no better than using each alone. This result is atypical, however. Patients who report no response to naphazoline have little change in rCBF after administration of this agent.

It thus may be possible, at least in certain situations, that decreases in rCBF do not cause worsening of symptoms, just as increases in rCBF do not necessarily produce improvement. In the case of naphazoline, NO may be released which could have a local or regional neuronal, or glial, effect on neurotransmission, but the vasodilatory properties of NO could be overshadowed by vasoconstrictive substances released concomitantly, which may or may not affect patient symptom report. Sensations resembling migraine auras are occasionally experienced after naphazoline instillation, perhaps reflecting its vasoconstrictive action. A novel therapeutic approach would be the topical ophthalmic use of nitroglycerin or other nitrovasodilators, currently being investigated in the treatment of glaucoma.[20]

REFERENCES

1. Goadsby PJ, Kauge H, Hoskin KL. Nitric oxide synthesis couples cerebral blood flow and metabolism. *Brain Res* 595: 167-170, 1992.

2. Regidor J, Edvinsson, Divac I. NOS neurons lie near branchings of cortical arterioles. *NeuroReport* 4: 112-114, 1993.

3. Appenzeller O. Pathogenesis of migraine. *Med Clin N Amer* 75(3): 763-789, 1991.

4. Morris R, Southam E, Gittins SR, Garthwaite J. NADPH-diaphorase staining in autonomic and somatic ganglia of the rat. *NeuroReport* 4: 62-64, 1993.

5. Iadecola C, Faris PL, Hartman BK, Xu X. Localization of NADPH diaphorase in neurons of the rostral ventral medulla; possible role of nitric oxide in central autonomic regulation and chemoreception. *Brain Res* 603: 173-179, 1993.

6. Edvisson L, MacKenzie ET, McCulloch J, Uddman R. Perivascular Innervation and Receptor Mechanisms in Cerebrovascular Bed. In: Wood JH (ed.). *Cerebral Blood Flow: Physiologic and Clinical Aspects*. New York: McGraw-Hill, 1987.

7. Nozaki K, Moskowitz MA, Maynard KI, Koketsu N, Dawson TM, Bredt DS, Snyder SH. Possible origins and distribution of immunoreactive nitric oxide synthase-containing nerve fibers in cerebral arteries. *J Cereb Blood Flow Metab* 13: 70-79, 1993.

8. Peticlerc E, Abel S, de Blois D, Poubelle PE, Marceau F. Effects of inter-leukin-1 receptor antagonist on three types of responses to interleukin-1 in rabbit isolated blood vessels. *J Cardiovasc Pharmacol* 19: 821-829, 1992.

9. Matsui TA, Takuwa Y, Johshita H, Yamashita K, Asano T. Possible role of protein kinase C-dependent smooth muscle contraction in the pathogenesis of chronic cerebral vasospasm. *J Cereb Blood Flow Metab* 11: 143-149, 1991.

10. Uddman R, Goadsby PJ, Jansen I, Edvinsson L. PACAP, a VIP-like pep-tide: immunohistochemical localization and effect upon cat pial arteries and cere-bral blood flow. *J Cereb Blood Flow Metab* 13: 291-297, 1993.

11. MacFarlane MS, Tasdemiroglu E, Moskowitz MA, Uemura Y, Wei EP, Kontos HA. Chronic trigeminal ganglionectomy or topical capsaicin application to pial vessels attenuates postocclusive cortical hyperemia but does not influence postischemic hypoperfusion. *J Cereb Blood Flow Metab* 11: 261-271, 1991.

12. Marinis MD, Fraioli B, Esposito V, Gagliardi FM, Agnoli A. Unilateral reduction of head pain and facial vasodilatation after Gasserian ganglion lesion. *Arch Neurol* 50: 203-208, 1993.

13. Jaanus SD, Pagano VT, Bartlett JD. Drugs affecting the autonomic ner-vous system. In: Bartlett JD, Jaanus SD (eds.). *Clinical Ocular Pharmacology.* Boston: Butterworth, 1989.

14. Hakim AM, Hogan MJ. In vivo binding of nimodipine in the brain: I. The effect of focal cerebral ischemia. *J Cereb Blood Flow and Metab* 11: 762-770, 1991.

15. Goldstein JA. *Chronic Fatigue Syndrome: The Struggle for Health.* Los Angeles: Chronic Fatigue Syndrome Institute, 1990.

16. Beer NA, Jakubowicz DJ, Beer RM, Arocha IR, Nestler JE. Effects of ni-trendipine on glucose tolerance and serum insulin and dehydroepiandrosterone sulfate levels in insulin-resistant obese and hypertensive men. *J Clin Endocrinol Metab* 76(1): 178-183, 1993.

17. Alborch E, Salom JB, Perales AJ, Torregrosa G, Miranda FJ, Alabadi JA, Jover T. Comparison of the anticonstrictor action of dihydropyridines (nimodi-pine and nicardipine) and Mg^{++} in isolated human cerebral arteries. *Eur J Phar-macol* 229: 83-89, 1992.

18. Blattner LA, Wier WG. Nitric oxide decreases < CA2 < *I in vascular smooth muscle by a CGMP dependent inhibition of calcium current (meeting abstr.). *Biophys J* 64(2): A217, 1993.

19. Triggle CR, Adeagbo ASO. Modulation of alpha-adrenoceptor-mediated responses by VSM-derived nitric oxide (NO) in rat isolated aortic rings (meeting abstr.). *FASEB J* 7(3): A336, 1993.

20. Nathanson JA. Nitrovasodilators as a new class of ocular hypotensive agents. *J Pharmacol Exp Ther* 260(3): 956-965, 1992.

Index

Abdominal pain, 102
Acetazolamide, 158,165,230
N-Acetyl-cysteine, 177,206
Acroparesthesias, 62
ACTH, 17,18,20,147
    in interferon therapy, 135
    response to corticotropin
        releasing hormone, 142
    stimulation by interleukin-1,
        19,134
    stimulation tests, 44,75,113
Acupuncture, 171,172
Adamantan compounds, 141,228-
    229
Adenosine triphosphate levels
    in CFS, 41
Adnexal masses, 102
Adrenal gland, 142,143,145
    in depression, 193
    in stress response, 17,44,143
α-Adrenergic blocking drugs, 103,
    104
β-Adrenergic blocking drugs, 101
α-Adrenergic receptors on platelets,
    19,80
Agent X, as possible causative
    agent, 5,20
Agnosias, 51
Agoraphobia, 49,54,106,158,159
Alcohol intolerance, 56,80-81
Allergies, 196,205
    nasal, 68-69,99,198,199
Alopecia, 99
Alprazolam, 153,158-159,227
Alternative CFS treatments, 129,
    177-179
Amantadine, 141,228
Amino acids, excitatory, 47,160,
    162,201

levels in CFS, 162,165,209,222
gamma-aminobutyric acid, 146-
    147,201
gamma-aminobutyric acid
    receptors, 201
    chloride channels in, 201
    ethanol affecting, 80-81
    interleukin-1 affecting, 111-
        112
    neurosteroids affecting, 74,
        138-139
    and interleukin-1 secretion, 134
Ampligen, 120,177,230
    antiviral activity of, 87,97,131,
        168,199
    in cognitive dysfunction, 87,168
    in depression, 135,152
    discontinuation of, 200
    as immunomodulatory agent, 12,
        41,87,97,131,191
    and interleukin-1 levels, 43,198,
        230
Amygdala, 24,34-35,173
    in depression, 114
    in limbic system, 24,33,143
    in memory, 24,32
    in post-traumatic stress disorder,
        143
    in respiratory abnormalities, 77
Anesthesia, effects in CFS patients,
    81
Anti-inflammatory drugs,
    nonsteroidal, 147
Antibiotic therapy, 132-133
Antidepressants, 12,153,225-226,
    227
    augmentation with thyroid
        hormones, 156,193,227
    mechanism of action, 170,201